WORK DISCUSSION

Tavistock Clinic Series

Margot Waddell (Series Editor)

Published by Karnac Books

Other titles in the Tavistock Clinic Series

Acquainted with the Night: Psychoanalysis and the Poetic Imagination, *edited by Hamish Canham & Carole Satyamurti*

Assessment in Child Psychotherapy, *edited by Margaret Rustin & Emanuela Quagliata*

Borderline Welfare: Feeling and Fear of Feeling in Modern Welfare, *by Andrew Cooper & Julian Lousada*

Creating New Families: Therapeutic Approaches to Fostering, Adoption, and Kinship Care, *edited by Jenny Kenrick, Caroline Lindsey, & Lorraine Tollemache*

Facing It Out: Clinical Perspectives on Adolescent Disturbance, *edited by Robin Anderson & Anna Dartington*

Inside Lives: Psychoanalysis and the Growth of the Personality, *by Margot Waddell*

Internal Landscapes and Foreign Bodies: Eating Disorders and Other Pathologies, *by Gianna Williams*

Looking into Later Life: A Psychoanalytic Approach to Depression and Dementia in Old Age, *edited by Rachael Davenhill*

Mirror to Nature: Drama, Psychoanalysis, and Society, *by Margaret Rustin & Michael Rustin*

Multiple Voices: Narrative in Systemic Family Psychotherapy, *edited by Renos K. Papadopoulos & John Byng-Hall*

Oedipus and the Couple, *edited by Francis Grier*

Organization in the Mind: Psychoanalysis, Group Relations, and Organizational Consultancy, *by David Armstrong, edited by Robert French*

Psychoanalysis and Culture: A Kleinian Perspective, *edited by David Bell*

Psychotic States in Children, *edited by Margaret Rustin, Maria Rhode, Alex Dubinsky, & Hélène Dubinsky*

Reason and Passion: A Celebration of the Work of Hanna Segal, *edited by David Bell*

Reflecting on Reality: Psychotherapists at Work in Primary Care, *edited by John Launer, Sue Blake, & Dilys Daws*

Sent Before My Time: A Child Psychotherapist's View of Life on a Neonatal Intensive Care Unit, *by Margaret Cohen*

Surviving Space: Papers on Infant Observation, *edited by Andrew Briggs*

The Anorexic Mind, *by Marilyn Lawrence*

The Learning Relationship: Psychoanalytic Thinking in Education, *edited by Biddy Youell*

The Many Faces of Asperger's Syndrome, *edited by Maria Rhode & Trudy Klauber*

Therapeutic Care for Refugees: No Place Like Home, *edited by Renos K. Papadopoulos*

Understanding Trauma: A Psychoanalytic Approach, *edited by Caroline Garland*

Unexpected Gains: Psychotherapy with People with Learning Disabilities, *edited by David Simpson & Lynda Miller*

"What Can the Matter Be?": Therapeutic Interventions with Parents, Infants, and Young Children, *edited by Louise Emanuel & Elizabeth Bradley*

Working Below the Surface: The Emotional Life of Contemporary Organizations, *edited by Clare Huffington, David Armstrong, William Halton, Linda Hoyle, & Jane Pooley*

Orders

Tel: +44 (0)20 7431 1075; Fax: +44 (0)20 7435 9076

Email: shop@karnacbooks.com

www.karnacbooks.com

WORK DISCUSSION

Learning from Reflective Practice in Work with Children and Families

Edited by

Margaret Rustin & Jonathan Bradley

Foreword by

Trudy Klauber

Routledge
Taylor & Francis Group
LONDON AND NEW YORK

First published 2008 by
Karnac Books

2 Park Square, Milton Park, Abingdon, Oxfordshire OX14 4RN
52 Vanderbilt Avenue, New York, NY 10017

Routledge is an imprint of the Taylor & Francis Group, an informa business

First issued in hardback 2019

British Library Cataloguing in Publication Data

A C.I.P. for this book is available from the British Library

ISBN: 978-1-85575-644-1 (pbk)
ISBN: 978-0-367-32985-3 (hbk)

Edited, designed, and produced by Communication Crafts

www.karnacbooks.com

CONTENTS

SERIES EDITOR'S PREFACE

Margot Waddell

Since it was founded in 1920, the Tavistock Clinic has developed a wide range of developmental approaches to mental health which have been strongly influenced by the ideas of psychoanalysis. It has also adopted systemic family therapy as a theoretical model and a clinical approach to family problems. The Clinic is now the largest training institution in Britain for mental health, providing postgraduate and qualifying courses in social work, psychology, psychiatry, and child, adolescent, and adult psychotherapy, as well as in nursing and primary care. It trains about 1,700 students each year in over 60 courses.

The Clinic's philosophy aims at promoting therapeutic methods in mental health. Its work is based on the clinical expertise that is also the basis of its consultancy and research activities. The aim of this Series is to make available to the reading public the clinical, theoretical, and research work that is most influential at the Tavistock Clinic. The Series sets out new approaches in the understanding and treatment of psychological disturbance in children, adolescents, and adults, both as individuals and in families.

No volume could better describe the work method that underpins the learning, thinking, training, and researching that goes on at the Tavistock than this account of the nature and culture of what has become known as "work discussion". Explored here in great detail is the method and application of this very particular approach, one based on a distinction that has become central to much of the Clinic's attitude to teaching and learning. The emphasis is not so much on the acquisition of knowledge and information as such—"a learning about" model—as on learning from experience. This latter brings together a combination of close observation of, and personal and interpersonal responses to, the minutiae of the work setting and its dynamics, both internal and external. Such a model depends on the development of hard-won capacities, and the descriptions offered here, both by students and by experienced staff, fully demonstrate the immense relevance of the approach, both to training and to a wide variety of work situations.

The book first outlines the process of the method itself, followed by descriptions of a range of settings, both in Britain and abroad, in which that method has been successfully applied. The contributors draw on experiences across age, culture, and race in, for example, schools, hospitals, residential homes, in a prison, and in a refugee community. The final chapter explores the implications of work discussion for research and policy-making more generally. Many of the situations narrated here are extreme, whether in terms of disturbance or of vulnerability, but these pages offer often moving insights into how effective the method can be and how truly impressive a developmental model it provides.

ACKNOWLEDGEMENTS

An enormous number of people have contributed to this book's coming into being, since the principal resource for the editors has been the work of many generations of work discussion seminar members and leaders. We wish to thank them all for their inspiration and for the many particular examples we have included in the book. The rich archive of material from the Tavistock Psycho-analytic Observational Studies course has been accessed with the help of Sara Riley and her team of course administrators, whose patience we have much appreciated. Particular thanks are also due to Christine Porter (for help with the work described by Suzanne Pabot), Sebastian Kraemer, Margot Waddell for her sustaining encouragement and detailed involvement as overall Series Editor, and to Caroline Weaver for her exceptional work in preparing the manuscript for publication, without which it would not have been possible to bring the project to completion.

Formal acknowledgement for permission to reprint versions of previously published papers is due to the *Journal of Child Psychotherapy* (Vol. 34, No. 1, April 2008) for Emil Jackson's chapter, to the editor of the *International Journal of Infant Observation* (Vol. 6, No. 2, April 2003) for Alison Hall's chapter, and to Phil Jones, editor of *Drama As Therapy: Theory, Practice and Research* (Routledge, 2007), for some material in Elizabeth Nixon's chapter.

The writers of individual chapters have responded with thoughtfulness, grace, and much hard work to our many editorial suggestions, which has made the editorial work very rewarding.

Finally, our greatest thanks are due to the children, young people, and families, and their workers, whose stories are at the heart of the book. Of course, all names have been changed and all individual identities have been made anonymous for publication, but we believe the book's value lies in the particularity of the experiences recounted.

We hope we have done justice to the human complexities that are the book's origin and *raison d'être*.

Margaret Rustin and Jonathan Bradley

ABOUT THE EDITORS AND CONTRIBUTORS

SERENELLA ADAMO SERPIERI is a child psychotherapist; she works as a psychologist in the Department of Mental Health in Naples and in private practice. She collaborates with the University of Naples "Federico II" in teaching and research activities. She is external examiner of two Tavistock/University of East London courses and a member of AIPPI (Italian Association of Child Psychotherapy) and of EFPP.

SIMONETTA M. G. ADAMO is full professor of clinical psychology at the University of Milan "Bicocca". She is a child and adolescent psychotherapist, member of the Tavistock Society of Psychotherapists, and co-organizer of the course "Working with Disruptive Adolescents" held at the Tavistock. She has planned and organized several educational projects in difficult contexts. Among others, she is responsible for all the psychological interventions in a project for adolescent dropouts, the Chance Project, run in Naples. Her main areas of interest and research are infant and young child observation, counselling with young people, psychoanalytically oriented work in paediatric wards, and emotional aspects in teaching and learning relationships.

FADUMO OSMAN AHMED currently works as a mental health practitioner and an assistant therapist at the Tavistock Child and Family Department. From October 2008 she will be working as a child psychotherapist in training with a learning and complex disability team.

KATIE ARGENT is a child and adolescent psychotherapist working in the Child and Family Department at the Tavistock Clinic. She works in the Refugee Team and is Chair of the Refugee Workshop; she manages the Tavistock Outreach in Primary Schools project with a clinical base in a primary school; she is course organizer for the Counselling in Educational Settings professional training; and she is joint convenor of the Groups Workshop.

JONATHAN BRADLEY is a consultant child and adolescent psychotherapist in the Adolescent Department, where he is the Child Psychotherapy Head. He is the Organising Tutor of the PG Dip/MA in Psychoanalytic Studies offered by the Tavistock Clinic and the University of East London. A two-year Work Discussion Seminar has always played a prominent part in this large course. He has written a number of books with the general reader in mind: *Understanding Your Ten Year Old Child; Understanding 15–17 Year Olds;* and *Coping With Life* (addressed specifically to adolescents). He is the Editor of the revised *Understanding Your Child* series, published by Jessica Kingsley. He is interested in the processes involved in group learning, and he has worked as a staff member in group relations events, both at the Tavistock and at the Leicester Conference.

MARGHERITA CASTELLANI is a trainee child psychotherapist at the Tavistock Clinic. Her earlier education was in the history of art in New York and London.

KARL FOSTER works as a creative practitioner in museums, galleries, schools, and other learning venues across the country. This work ranges from museum interpretation to design work, project development, and public commissions.

PAOLA GIUSTI is a child psychotherapist; she works as a psychologist in a Child and Adolescent Unit in Naples and in private practice. She collaborates with the University of Naples "Federico II" in teaching and research activities and is also a member of the AIPPI (Italian Association of Child Psychotherapy) and of the EFPP.

ALISON HALL is a paediatric oncology/haematology outreach nurse specialist, based in Yorkhill Hospital, Glasgow. She has worked in children's nursing for almost the past two decades, and for most of that time she has specialized in children's cancer nursing.

STUART HANNAH is a social worker and child and adolescent psychotherapist trained at the Tavistock Clinic. His career started at the Cotswold Community, where he became interested in the psychodynamics of individuals, groups, and organizations. He has since worked in a variety of inner-city social-work settings and the Adolescent Department of the Tavistock. He now works as a child psychotherapist in the Pebbles Therapeutic Community in South Essex and in private practice.

CLAUDIA HENRY is a child and adolescent psychotherapist currently working in Harlow CAMHS. Prior to training as a child psychotherapist, Claudia worked for a number of years as a hospital play specialist in a large paediatric hospital. She also spent part of her clinical training working in a hospital on a neonatal intensive care unit.

EMIL JACKSON is a consultant child and adolescent psychotherapist working at the Tavistock Clinic and Brent Centre for Young People. In addition to clinical work, Emil is involved in teaching on a number of courses at the Tavistock and is Assistant Organising Tutor for the Child Psychotherapy training. Over the past 10 years he has been involved in developing and managing a range of outreach mental health projects in schools within which work discussion groups for staff have been the cornerstone.

TRUDY KLAUBER is a Consultant Child and Adolescent Psychotherapist who originally trained as a secondary teacher. She is Dean of Postgraduate Studies at the Tavistock and Portman NHS Foundation Trust. Her interests include working with parents, clinical supervision, and teaching and developing access to high-quality training for all sectors of the mental health, public, and voluntary sector workforce. She teaches in the United Kingdom, in Italy, and, occasionally, in the United States and has published a number of papers about clinical work with parents and children and young people with autism, Asperger's syndrome, and a variety of applications of psychoanalytic thinking.

SHEILA MILLER is a consultant child psychotherapist in the Tavistock Child & Family Department, and she led Work Discussion Seminars for many years on the Observational Studies Course. From 1994 to 2001 she lived and worked in South Africa, where she collaborated with colleagues in using and adapting the Tavistock model of Work Discussion and Infant Observation seminars.

ELIZABETH NIXON worked for many years as a drama therapist specializing in work with children and young people with learning disabilities. She subsequently also trained as a child and adolescent psychotherapist.

SUSANNAH ELISABETH PABOT holds an MA in children's literature and has worked as a London-based journalist specializing in the children's book market. Whilst studying on the Observation Course at the Tavistock Clinic, she spent two years in a London infant school in the position of learning mentor. She now lives in Paris, France, where she works as a freelance writer and editor.

MARGARET RUSTIN is a consultant child and adolescent psychotherapist at the Tavistock Clinic, London, where she has been Head of Child Psychotherapy since 1986. She has pioneered and supported the extension of training in psychoanalytic observational approaches to training across the United Kingdom and in a number of other countries. She has co-authored, with Michael Rustin, *Narratives of Love and Loss* and *Mirror to Nature* and has co-edited *Closely Observed Infants*, as well as *Psychotic States in Children* and *Assessment in Psychotherapy*.

MICHAEL RUSTIN is professor of sociology at the University of East London and a visiting professor at the Tavistock Clinic. He is an Honorary Affiliate Member of the British Psychoanalytic Society and is the author of *The Good Society and the Inner World* and *Reason and Unreason*, among other works.

SUZAN SAYDER trained as a child and adolescent psychotherapist at the Tavistock & Portman NHS Foundation Trust. She is currently employed by the Tavistock Clinic and Brent Centre for Young People to do outreach work at two secondary comprehensive schools in London, with both pupils and staff groups. She also works in the Brent Centre family service. In addition, she teaches on Tavistock courses.

RITA TAMAJO CONTARINI is a child psychotherapist; she works as a psychologist in a Child and Adolescent Unit in Naples and in private practice. She collaborates with the University of Naples "Federico II" in teaching and research activities and is a member of AIPPI (Italian Association of Child Psychotherapy) and of the EFPP.

GIANNA WILLIAMS was Organising Tutor of the Course in Psychoanalytic Observational Studies for over 20 years and has taught work discussion seminars both in England and abroad since the early 1970s. She founded several Tavistock Model Courses in Psychoanalytic Observational Studies and in Child Psychotherapy in European and Latin American countries. She is currently teaching on the Tavistock Doctorate in Child Psychotherapy and works as a psychoanalyst in private practice.

GARY YEXLEY currently works as Director of the therapeutic community featured in his chapter. As part of the charity Childhood First (formally the Peper Harow Foundation), his team specializes in the residential treatment of children and young people who have suffered long-term relational and abusive trauma. He includes work discussion seminars in his programme of support and training for staff, as part of a university-accredited course designed in collaboration with the Tavistock Centre.

FOREWORD

Trudy Klauber

It is an honour to be asked to write the foreword to a book that sets out the history, theory, and practice of work discussion as developed at the Tavistock Clinic.

In a very powerful way, the Tavistock Clinic has always been in the business of developing a model for learning that enhances the worker's capacity, whatever his or her role and task. Currently, this links in a coherent way with policies developed in the Department of Health and the Department for Children, Schools and Families for "creating capable teams" and individuals whose *skills for health, social care, or justice* are required across an entire workforce. The Tavistock Clinic has been striving to do this since it was founded just after the First World War. Over the years, its commitment to improving mental health has always meant that training people has been as important as the clinical work itself. The training has always been designed to ensure that people take what they have learnt with them to their various roles, wherever they work.

The work discussion model is the epitome of the application of psychoanalytic ideas. It owes much to some extraordinary individuals who worked at the Tavistock Clinic before, during, and after the Second World War. In the 1930s, Wilfred Bion was trying to understand groups and was later involved, with John Rickman and others, in developing effective methods for British Army officer selection. They used leaderless groups to see who would emerge with enough ability to keep thinking, not too interested in power but, rather, in using *authority* and able to keep in mind other people's needs and skills. John Bowlby, who later went on to develop and research his attachment theory, observed evacuees and other children in the Hampstead Nurseries of Anna Freud. James and Joyce Robertson filmed children in brief separation—films that made a significant contribution to the general understanding of children's experience and the impact of sudden loss and the trauma of inadequate substitute care. Michael Balint was working with GPs in small groups discussing their work, and Esther Bick was offering infant observation seminars from the late 1940s. The individuals I have mentioned—and there are many more—created a rich culture of inquiry and thoughtfulness and applied their exceptional minds to evolving ways of using groups for study, to discuss work, and to understand group and organizational dynamics.

Over time, Martha Harris, who developed the Child Psychotherapy training at the Tavistock, created a new method of training: the work discussion seminar, which proved to be a powerful teaching and learning experience. It took shape in her capable and creative hands and has since then spread to become an integral part of very many of the Tavistock Clinic's large portfolio of courses (see Margaret Rustin's chapter 1, on historical and theoretical perspectives, in this volume.)

It seems that there was a particular *zeitgeist* that allowed for the evolution of such a teaching tool, which is applicable in relation to *any* work situation involving human interaction. The model recognizes the worker's own expertise and attempts, through the group's work and the help of a psychoanalytically trained seminar leader, to add something extra. This difficult-to-define additional something has an immense impact on people. It strengthens their capacity to struggle to work effectively—perhaps one dares to say therapeutically—in often very difficult, distressing, and challenging work situations (which, one should say, are mostly non-clinical).

The experience of being part of a work discussion seminar is one of the elements to which former students allude as something that has *changed their lives*. They feel that it is something special (see the comment by a former student quoted at the end of Jonathan Bradley's chapter 2, this volume.)

Two very experienced consultant child and adolescent psychiatrists have separately spoken to me about the profound impact of the Tavistock Work Discussion model on them and on their professional development. The first impact for both of them was that they felt disturbed, even provoked. In fact, in my experience it is not at all uncommon for students not to like the seminar much to start with. Both of the psychiatrists remembered the discomfort they felt in the early seminars when the leader did not offer didactic teaching and did not actively lead the group into particular lines of discussion, asking the group, instead, to voice the thoughts that had occurred as they had listened to the presenter reading his or her account of an interaction from the workplace. They were struck and inspired by the culture of curiosity and inquiry and by the absence of a rush towards conclusions and solutions in action. Both have continued to feel that, within themselves, they developed a much greater sense of openness and of having the patience and humility to allow something to unfold, as it so often did in the course of the seminar. Perhaps most of all, they were appreciative of having had the experience of something that characterizes a truly reflective state of mind.

The work discussion model depends on participants being encouraged simply to "tell it like it is". It is often a very new experience for people to be encouraged to write in the first person and to include subjective thoughts and, sometimes, some acutely painful, troubling feelings. The atmosphere of acceptance and genuine interest gradually rubs off. Indeed, in well-led seminars it might be more accurate to say that the individuals in the group begin to identify with the seminar leader's capacities and way of working.

Bion's concept of containment, which is mentioned recurrently throughout this book, is one way of describing the establishment of a setting that is accepting but not passive, thought-provoking without being directly challenging, and inclusive without making everyone seem to be saying or thinking the same thing. If this is achieved, then something transformative can happen. Students from a range of health, education, and social care agencies say that work discussion changes the way they think about their work. It may or may not change their practice in overt ways, but it certainly changes the way they think about their client group, their task, and their own contribution to the interpersonal dynamics that cause so much of what is commonly known as "work-related stress" or "burn-out".

To my mind, the strength of the work discussion model is that the change within the worker really is a transformation. Participants can look at details they had not noticed previously. They can begin to appreciate that projected feeling has a reality that can be useful if seen as potential communication. When people feel very disturbed, upset, or angry, for example, the feelings are transmitted to those around them.

We all recognize this in ordinary life when we witness "incidents" in the street, on buses, or at community events. A very angry or agitated person might be looking for a fight with someone, or might be very frightened of attack—or both. The work discussion model expressly includes the concept of projection—studying the way feelings get into the worker and may, indeed, stir up the members of the seminar group when they are paying attention to a detailed narrative.

The thinking in seminars about what happens, what is said, and what is picked up in feeling states is one of the additional ingredients that acts to free group members from feeling responsible for everything, from feeling *no good* at their job, and from reacting impulsively. This is modelled in the group and by the seminar leader—as you will read in most of the chapters in this book. Perhaps it is this that really allows that overused word "empathy" to become something real. The group can begin to feel for each other and for the people described in presentations—and, if the leader can struggle with sticking to the task, they can begin to see the possibility of having a reflective space in their own minds when they are at work. This is a surprisingly powerful element in their being able to provide clients with a sense of a different kind of interaction and of the possibility of not endlessly repeating entrenched patterns of thought or behaviour.

This book brings into the public domain a timely collection of essays describing a method of teaching, of group supervision, and of peer-group thinking that has an extraordinarily creative and vital impact both on workers and on the work they do.

INTRODUCTION

Margaret Rustin

This book aims to describe the evolution and contemporary practice of work discussion in relation to a wide range of professional work with children, adolescents, and families. It is the editors' hope to provide a historical and theoretical perspective and an engrossing and challenging sequence of case studies that exemplify the nature of the learning process and the deeper quality of engagement with the work task that work discussion makes possible.

At times, a suitable alternative title for the book seemed to be "Studies in Containment", since the concept of containment proved to be so central as we explored the archives of students' work discussion papers to gain a sense of the spread of possible contributions. As noted in the first and final chapters, the theoretical power of Bion's concept has proved far-reaching. Its applicability and relevance in an enormous variety of contexts is what struck us repeatedly. Bion's core insight was to understand the dynamic interplay of "container" and "contained" with respect to emotional experience. The "container" is his term for the more mature mind (the mother in Bion's account of early psychic development), which has the capacity for observation, reflection, and, ultimately, transformation of elements of emotional experience that have not yet reached meaningful shape or representation at the level of verbal thought. The "contained" is the less developed mind (the infant, in Bion's model), which lacks sophisticated capacities for thinking and expression and requires a relationship with a container in order to develop mental capacities for thinking, communication, and judgement. The interplay between the two is via conscious and unconscious verbal and non-verbal communication, including, especially, the form of communication defined as "projective identification". This is registered through the mental reverie (openness to receive primitive emotional communication) of the mother/container and acquires meaning through the response generated by this communication. So, in the early months, it is the parental responsiveness to the baby's somatic communications that gradually allows distinctions to be made between pain, hunger, loneliness, anxiety, tiredness, and so on. The baby thus comes to know and understand himself through being known. Bion suggested that this model of development was central to the therapeutic potential of psychoanalysis. In this book it will become evident, we think, how very powerfully the model describes an essential aspect of relationships between professional workers and their clients. Many of the chapters record the dawning realization of workers about what was required of them to become an effective container and what were the painful emotions they had to get to know in this process.

We have organized the book in four sections. The first provides an overview of the background and scope of current practice. It includes chapters addressing the viewpoints of seminar leader and student, and also one that suggests the enormous potential for development of the paradigm within many institutions whose staff could be supported in difficult work by having opportunities for ongoing discussion of their work.

The second—and longest—section provides a remarkably vivid demonstration of work discussion in action. The chapters are all based on accounts by students who have attended work discussion seminars in the context of Master's level courses that focus on the development of students' observational skills within a psychoanalytic framework and their application to ongoing professional work. The chapters are grouped under three headings: one about work in educational contexts, one in health settings, and one linked to varieties of social care. The range of professions represented is wide: drama therapist, learning mentor, teaching assistant, creative artist, hospital play-worker, children's cancer nurse, therapeutic children's home worker, community refugee worker, prison crèche worker, residential social worker. This mixture seems quite characteristic of the range of people who seek out this kind of course, and it could well have included others, such as speech and language therapists, art therapists, psychologists, housing officers, school nurses, Sure Start workers, adolescent inpatient nursing assistants, and so on. Interestingly, the prior background of the student group is even more varied. Such courses attract people exploring possible career change and have included journalists, lawyers, writers, academics, and head teachers, as well as people with little prior educational experience whose natural talent for human relationships has drawn them to undertake study of this sort.

These chapters are quite varied in their level of complexity and sophistication, but we think they all give evidence of the process of learning that work discussion has set in motion. In this respect, the range of individuals who might be encountered in any work discussion seminar are well represented by the selection included in this volume. Some of them are writing about fresh and unfamiliar experiences and reaching for a language adequate to describe what they see and do and what happens to their understanding and perception. Others are making bold efforts to integrate the idea of observation and the concepts of psychoanalysis with a previous theoretical schema. This leads, at times, to a sense of a much-changed professional identity, and sometimes to most original formulations. This kind of writing powerfully conveys what it is like to be part of a work discussion seminar, where ideas take shape quite gradually but with a marked sense of discovery and excitement. The extreme level of pain and anxiety that workers face with some of their clients and the degree of self-questioning about their role, about institutions, and about human possibilities that they can be encouraged to open up to is also well documented in this section of the book.

The third section looks at some examples of adaptation of the work discussion model in international projects. Here, again, the flexibility of the approach is evident: useful for workers with little training in a very deprived, traumatized community in South Africa, in a sophisticated multilayered community intervention and research project in Naples, and in an unusual children's home in Mexico. Work discussion has travelled well and is much used in courses similar to the ones we have drawn from in many countries, but the chapters included in the international section all describe ways in which the model can be developed in innovative ways within particular projects. These chapters therefore also serve to suggest the creative potential of work discussion and give evidence of how meaningful and enabling it proves to be in a variety of contexts.

In the fourth part and the final chapter, there is a discussion of the wider implications of this educational practice: its research potential, its policy relevance, and its location within the development of public sector services. This chapter brings to mind myriads of possible projects and lines of enquiry.

We believe the book will be valuable not only to past and current students and teachers of work discussion, but to a very much wider professional public concerned to think about the quality of work done in educational, health, and social care settings and the urgent task of sustaining and developing workers' professional capacities in difficult contexts. Burn-out is a serious problem in many professions, and nowhere more so than social work and teaching. We think that the method we describe of reflecting on experience is a potent source of renewal and growth of capacity.

PART I

WORK DISCUSSION: AN OVERVIEW

CHAPTER ONE

Work discussion: some historical and theoretical observations

Margaret Rustin

Despite its rather prosaic and literal nomenclature, work discussion as a component of professional education and practice has flourished in varied contexts since it began to figure as a systematic element in advanced training courses in the mid- and late 1960s. This chapter attempts to elucidate where the concept came from and discusses its significance. Although there has been an expanding literature on psychoanalytic infant observation (for example, Briggs, 2002; Miller, Rustin, Rustin, & Shuttleworth, 1989; Reid, 1997) and its later observational derivatives—young child observation, observation of the elderly (Davenhill, Balfour, & Rustin, 2007), and institutional observation (Hinshelwood & Skogstad, 2000) being particularly important developments—there has not, as yet, been a parallel growth in writing about work discussion. Perhaps its unglamorous name has had something to do with this, but probably more significant is the way in which it can disappear as a distinctive category and become subsumed under more familiar educational activities: it is easily placed as part of the now widespread notion of "reflective practice", and much of it can be relabelled as "clinical supervision". However, quite a lot is lost if the particular meaning that work discussion originally had is put aside, and within many courses offering opportunities for professional development and now validated as postgraduate degrees it holds a central position.

The systematic discussion of experience of work with small and stable groups of professional workers is the kind of work discussion that this book describes. It addresses the particular place work discussion has had in health, education, and social care contexts, and the form it has taken in the study of a wide range of work with children, families, and young people. The methodology of this kind of experiential learning is explored from a number of perspectives in the opening section. The theoretical background is a belief in the central importance of the emotional dynamics of experience at work. This entails a focus on those feelings, both conscious and unconscious, evoked in the worker by the task, context, institutional constraints, and daily relationships.

Interest in the relevance of unconscious factors in understanding the nature of work has gained considerable currency in the last six decades. Seminal books such as *The Unconscious At Work* (Obholzer & Roberts, 1994) have popularized the idea of omnipresent beneath-the-surface phenomena that have to be studied if the explicit aims of any work practice are to be achieved. The ways in which unconscious emotional forces can disrupt and distort professional practice and its outcome have become an object of study, and the power of this insight is such that it has travelled widely—into institutional consultancy, forms of professional supervision, applied group relations, and a range of training approaches. This attention to the unconscious makes evident the psychoanalytic roots of this tradition, to which other theoretically relevant ideas from group psychology, systems theory, and cognitive and developmental science have been added in varying combinations. Within this much larger body of work, this volume on work discussion represents one line of development in a field within which, while there is much shared in common, there is also much that is distinctive in the different tributaries.

Work discussion and child psychotherapy

So what constitutes work discussion? The first work discussion seminars actually labelled as such were offered by the child psychotherapist and psychoanalyst Martha Harris to a mixed group of people interested in a broad way in psychoanalytic ideas: Some of them were going on to train as child psychotherapists, others wanted to apply psychoanalytic insights in their established professional contexts. There was a strong representation from the world of education, as the group included educational psychologists, teachers in special education (in schools known then as schools for "maladjusted" or "delicate" children), and teachers working in ILEA (Inner London Education Authority) primary schools that provided small groups for children who did not cope well in the classroom (the sort of groups that subsequently came to be called "nurture groups"). There was also an art therapist, a social worker, and a paediatrician. The individuals had not met each other prior to the first seminar, and no one knew what was going to happen—except that they hoped to get help in understanding the children with whom they worked. They learnt that what was expected was that each of them, in turn, was to bring a detailed written account of something interesting or worrying from their experience at work. A few years later, Martha Harris wrote down the essence of what she wanted to provide for the course outline of the two-year psychoanalytic observational studies course that had gradually developed, which also included infant observation and psychoanalytic theory seminars. This is how she put it:

> Students bring detailed studies of their work for discussion in seminars. This enables a wider acquaintance to be obtained of the different settings in which children are cared for by professional workers. The studies presented include the interaction between the students themselves and their charges and in many cases pose questions about their role with colleagues in the organisation within which they are working. The presentation is then discussed by the rest of the group led by a seminar-leader experienced in work with children and adolescents, although not necessarily in the particular context within which the presenter is working.
>
> No particular technique is taught in these seminars. The members are encouraged to consider and to discuss appropriate ways of dealing with the situations and material described after their possible meanings have been explored.
>
> The aim of the seminar is to sharpen perceptions and to enhance the exercise of imagination so that a richer understanding of the personality interactions described may ensue, on the basis of evidence of motivation springing from internal unconscious sources. Education in sensitivity and increased awareness is a gradual process, inevitably attended by some degree of anxiety. "Not noticing" is one outcome of the defences against experiencing psychic pain in oneself and others. Becoming able to approach it more closely, and also coming to terms with the fact that there are no experts able to offer instant solutions is one of the problems with which each student in these seminars has to cope, to some extent. Likewise for

> the seminar leader it can be a continual exercise to struggle with his feelings of inadequacy in carrying the parental role attributed to him and to do the best that he can from his own experience to throw some additional light on the situation presented.

The points made in this brief but evocative description point to the theoretical origins of this methodology and raise many issues for discussion. They include the emphasis on detailed reports from the workplace, on the range of professional settings represented in a seminar group, on the role and responsibilities of the worker, on the worker's relationships with both children and colleagues at work, and on the ubiquity of unconscious sources for many of the everyday interactions to be studied. In particular, the idea is mooted that unconscious motivation will be part of the worker's input to the interactions and not only something to be studied in the behaviour of the children.

The history and intellectual origins of work discussion

Before considering these themes further, our focus needs to widen its scope to investigate the influences shaping the work discussion concept deployed here. The 1960s climate of educational and social change—comprehensive schools, the widening of higher education and the Plowden report on primary education, for example—is an important backdrop. Interest in the idea of intergenerationally transmitted cycles of deprivation had had such an impact at policy levels that the Tavistock Clinic and the Tavistock Institute of Human Relations were provided with a new building within which clinical services for NHS patients and research and consultative work could develop. The optimism of the time ran quite deep—the democratization of the insights of psychoanalysis was an evident component of the concept of work discussion, since it operated on the basis that people of very varied levels of professional status and experience could learn from each other and also assumed that the unconscious could be explored not only on the psychoanalytic couch but also through free group discussion of emotionally significant events from the workplace.

The Tavistock Clinic and Institute housed some very original thinkers in the post-war period, and some of their ideas were vital to the generation of work discussion methodology. At the broadest level was the ambition to influence community mental health through interventions at many different levels, including the workplace. The early work of Elliot Jaques and the research studies of Isabel Menzies

Lyth and her colleagues demonstrated how creative were the ideas of psychoanalysis about unconscious anxieties and defences when applied to social systems and institutions. Hugely influential also were the ideas on role, task, and organization of A. K. Rice and others, including Eric Miller, Pierre Turquet, and Robert Gosling, as well as the study of large and small group interactions and the establishment of a programme of Group Relations conferences to further this study. Senior figures at the Tavistock thus shared a conviction, growing from the work of W. R. Bion on group phenomena and the wartime and post-war application of some of these ideas, that group life could be understood and could have therapeutic and developmental potential. The pre-eminence of the much more private work of the analyst–patient pair was thus challenged by a lively sense of all that could be achieved by groups able to function as "work-groups" in Bion's definition. The work discussion group probably derived its name, in part, from Bion's valuing of the working potential of a group that is able to avoid falling into the "basic assumptions" of dependence, pairing, and fight/flight and to enlist, instead, the ego capacities of its members to tackle the agreed task, to become a "work-group".

A very important contribution to professional learning had also been made by Michael Balint (Balint, 1957), who invented a specific form of group learning for doctors (mostly general practitioners) usually subsequently referred to as "Balint groups".[1] These groups had a regular meeting time and an ongoing life and were, indeed, focused on the professional life and anxieties of the group members, who were invited to describe a case that was on their minds. They were not expected to prepare this beforehand: instead, Balint relied on the group ethos and process to elicit material that could lead to an investigation of difficulties in the doctor–patient relationship that were disturbing the doctor's professional capacities and decision making. This was a form of work discussion distinct from that described in this book because of its uni-professional group composition, its absence of written preparation, and its greater use of implicit or explicit interpretation of the worker's emotional experience.

However, what was the case from the mid-1960s onwards for some time was that staff at the Tavistock all had some experience of group life being an object of study. They might, as doctors, be members of a Balint group, or attend a "study group" that met over a period to study its own behaviour with a consultant, or go as a member to a Leicester Group Relations conference. They would also, if they were clinicians, be members of multidisciplinary teams where cases were discussed usually with a great deal of respect for the differing disciplinary viewpoints as well as hot debate over disagreements, and with an assumption that the most senior members of staff presented their clinical work for discussion as well as the junior staff undertaking training. Sometimes the group process was made use of in the understanding of the clinical phenomena of the case, so that "study-group" methodology and more traditional case conference discussion were integrated.

Some recent research into Tavistock history by Sebastian Kraemer (personal communication) has also drawn attention to another source for study group and work discussion methodology. He noted that Bion and Bowlby, the two intellectual giants of the Tavistock Clinic, had both been influenced by close relationships (both personal and professional) with Quakers, and he suggests that the circle of chairs that is the physical setting for this work in groups is an echo of the Quaker meeting. This is particularly pertinent in respect of study groups, where the consultant does not speak to start things off but waits for whatever may emerge, just as Quakers wait for the Spirit to be made manifest when someone is moved to speak. The work discussion group method is an important variant here, because there is a seminar leader with leadership responsibilities. In some adaptations of the model, there is a mixture of modalities: the leader may be called a facilitator or even consultant, and the work is approached in a less structured way than the one described here. These are important differences, since the closer one gets to a study group with its more therapeutic style, the further away one is from the idea that the group members are there to study their work role and to reflect on their experience at work in close detail, with the expectation that they can learn from this process and then apply their enlarged understanding in the work setting. However, it is useful to see the family resemblance between all of these forms of groups, particularly since individual group leaders vary in their approach, especially with respect to how much they may comment on the group's own functioning as a way of enabling difficult issues to be addressed.

All of this added up to great value being placed at the Tavistock on working in groups, but at the same time there was a very different lens suggested by infant observation. Esther Bick's invention of infant observation for the very first group of Tavistock child psychotherapy trainees in 1948 had been refined over time, and at its heart was the experience of a two-year weekly observation of a baby growing up from birth at home, in interaction with mother and with others in the home. A finely detailed account of all that could be recalled was written up as soon as possible after the hour-long observation had been concluded. This material was brought to a small weekly group of up to five people, each observing a baby. Members of the seminar each took a complete seminar to present their observations, and others then contributed their thoughts and feelings, with the seminar leader taking the role of weaving together what emerged to construct as rich as possible an account of the family relationships observed, the baby's developing personality, and the possible meanings of all that had taken place. This model of conducting a seminar was central to the evolution of work discussion. Pride of place was to be given to the material presented, and all details were seen as potentially significant. The group shared a gradually growing knowledge of each other's work settings and responsibilities, just as infant observers shared the process of getting to know each of the babies and families presented. Each member of the group was to be accorded an equal space, and their experience was given equal attention. The quality of the group's experience in the seminar depended on the careful preparation done by the presenter of the day, so there was a sense of camaraderie, especially important in the early months of the work when infant observers often found it very difficult to remember what they had seen and work discussion seminar members found it similarly difficult to make the focus of their writing-up one that would facilitate exploration. The task of noticing and noting in mind one's own behaviour while having to get on with the job, whatever it is, proves very challenging for most people, and to combine the reporting of verbal interaction and obvious activity with the more subtle description of private thoughts, atmosphere, pauses, facial expression, and bodily pose takes a good deal of practice.

The essence of the matter is the focus on observation and the expanding range of what is observed and recorded. This involves, for the worker, finding a part of the self able to step back a little from the immediate and keep an eye on both internal and external events, the inner workings of one's own conscious thoughts and fleeting sensations, and the events all around one in the interactions at work, which may involve quite a number of people. Of course the training in observation provided by the task of infant observation is enormously relevant for work discussion, and it is a simultaneous experience in many courses where students do both. The creative conjunction is also embedded in other courses (Briggs & Canham, 1999) that provide observational training of other sorts, such as institutional observation, alongside work discussion. Because the infant observer does not have to do anything other than observe, he or she can thus acquire an enhanced capability for observing detailed sequences. This background habit of close observation supports the worker trying to notice, think, and take action, often in quick sequence, and, indeed, in the seminars a very common occurrence is for the group to try to unpick—and slow down—the events by asking themselves about each step a little further.

Child observation and work discussion: an example

It may be useful at this point to provide an example of the sort of observations made and brought for discussion. The writer worked as a learning support assistant in a specialist day unit for primary-school-aged children. The link to infant observation is made explicit, and the physicality of the moment is very vividly described.

> My first impression of Simon, then aged 7, was that he physically appeared to fill the space. He is an overweight child with a round face, thick, short brown hair, and large brown eyes. His clothes are often too small for him and appear tight and uncomfortable. During my first day in the classroom, he seemed quite withdrawn and anxious, moving himself around awkwardly, flapping his hands, and rolling his eyes into the back of his head—quite a contrast from several of the other children who appeared uncontained in quite a different way: more aggressive, larger-than-life figures, full of anger.

Here is an extract from a recent observation in the classroom:

> Simon moved around the classroom seeming to spill out all over the place. He stood over the beanbag that he was aiming to land on and clumsily sat down, squashing Adam's feet as he landed. "Ow, Simon, get off my legs!" Adam shouted, nudging him hard with his elbow. Simon flinched and shouted "fuck off, stupid", appearing afraid and embarrassed at the tight squash and freed Adam's feet. Simon leaned over the container of books that was by his side and removed one and began flicking through its pages. He became fidgety and anxious and began scraping his back against the wall. He wriggled down, lay on his back, and held his legs up

> high into the air. This seemed to help ground him. Once again, he leaned awkwardly into Adam, who, to my surprise, ignored the discomfort. Simon opened up a page of the book and appeared to look at it for several minutes. The illustration was of a pig who had clearly got himself into a mess. "Look at the pig, look at the pig", Simon called out and flapped the pages into Adam's face. Adam pulled back, took a look, and found the illustration amusing. Simon watched to see Adam's reaction and then withdrew the book and continued to look through it before being asked to put it away.

The writer commented:

> This gave me some idea of how Simon was feeling, and I thought back to my infant observations and what Esther Bick describes when discussing the newborn in her paper entitled "The Experience of Skin in Early Object Relations" (1968). Simon seemed to be in such an unintegrated state, trying to hold himself together by creating a situation in which there was an equivalent of a continuous skin, with no gap, by fitting himself into a confined space and sliding to the floor. Simon then tried to communicate something about how bad he was feeling by showing Adam the picture of the pig—a large, rounded animal shaped like himself that was in a pickle.

The challenges of work discussion: disturbance of complacency and established practice

Now let us return to themes suggested by Martha Harris' description quoted earlier and explore their theoretical significance. The first thing that strikes anyone joining a work discussion seminar is the difficulty of the task of writing a detailed account of events at work. It sounds simple, but it is not. Centrally problematic is the implicit request not to define beforehand what was going on in the events reported. The details are to be observed, not selected so as to give weight to a particular line of thinking. The aim is to strive for a relatively theory-free and non-judgemental attitude to everyone involved, including oneself. The apparently meaningless is just as valuable in the record as the probably or obviously significant. The debt to the free-association method within psychoanalysis is an obvious one. There has to be enough background for people to be able to make sense of the context, but not so much as to deaden the impact of the immediate events in question, and not so many pages of description as to exhaust one's listeners.

The theoretical idea at the root of this demand that the writer should not already know the answer is the value psychoanalysts, and Bion in particular, place on being able to stay with the question, not rush to the answer. *Not* knowing is held to be a primary requirement of being able to "get to know" something. The distinction is between a form of "knowledge" that impedes exploration and learning because it is saturated knowledge, without space for discovery and an active relationship to the as yet unknown, and a process of cognitive and imaginative relating to experience that is a transitive and provisional one and leaves room for changing emotions and for uncertainty. The theory of work discussion as pedagogy is that the seminar leader's task is the creation and sustaining of an atmosphere of enquiry in the group characterized by curiosity, scepticism, fellow-feeling, debate, differences, so that the unknown can become less unwelcome and new thoughts, questions, and perceptions find fertile ground. There is not one "right" way to do or have done whatever is being studied: instead, there are some facts that can be viewed in many different ways, yielding new lines of enquiry.

This can be very far-reaching, since it can, for example, raise quite unexpected ideas and conflicts about what the role of a teacher or psychologist or social worker in fact is. The obvious—the starting point for each worker who already has a working model of what their job is about and an internal authority in the background felt to support this way of going about things—is the thing to be brought into question. This is, in fact, why work discussion in some form can—and perhaps should—be a career-long form of professional development. The whole point is the new perspective that can be embraced to enrich the familiar.

The decision to create groups mixed in terms of intellectual and professional background, differentiating the methodology from Balint's type of group, is intriguing. It was, no doubt, in part a consequence of the particular range of people who had expressed interest at that time in studying their experience at work from a psychoanalytic perspective, but it also seems to represent the commitment to learning from a plurality of sources. Just as infant observation seminars were to be stimulated by the differing familial worlds of the babies observed, so the work discussion group was to attempt to learn about the lives of children and young people in many contexts—school, playground, residential settings, community clinics, and so on—and the seminar members were also invited to absorb a sense of the many different professions involved in children's welfare and education. This professional pluralism went well beyond the traditional multidisciplinary mix of child guidance clinics, and perhaps prefigures the ideas that have become embedded in recent public policy about the necessity for joined-up thinking about children's development and for collaborative practice in the spheres of health, social care, and education. It was quite remarkably different from the dominant uni-disciplinary model of university education at that time and suggested, instead, that the mixing of modes of thought and vertices of observation was what could be most invigorating. It is interesting to note, in fact, that debates about teaching methods in education following on Basil Bernstein's differentiation between "collection" and "integrated" codes led to the theorization of a pedagogy (the "integrated" code) in which the concepts and theories used were more implicitly defined and learning was problem- or experience-based. This approach relied on the idea that learners could bring different perspectives to bear on the object of study. There was not one right definition, to be imparted by the teacher in a hierarchical relationship to the learners, but, instead, a more "horizontal" exchange of ideas. The professional pluralism of work discussion methods is an example of this kind of approach (Bernstein, 1975, especially Part II).

What distinguished the task of work discussion from infant observation was, most fundamentally, the twin focus of the recording of detailed interactions, with an emphasis on understanding the role of the worker and exploring its potential. The concept of role, and its link to a grasp of the nature and task of the organization in which the worker was embedded, introduced seminar members to thinking about organizational life and gave the seminar a social and at times political dimension. The tension between the psychoanalytic interest in the internal world and subjective meanings and the external work context, with its many demands and inherent limitations, was continually in play. Sometimes this would appear through different positions being espoused by different members of the seminar group, one wanting to prioritize the dynamic power of individual unconscious phantasy and another emphasizing external factors shaping behaviour. Debates about causation were rarely explicit, but the movement back and forth between perspectives could allow for the recognition of the ongoing influence in both directions. For example, the more primitive and often authoritarian forms of morality characteristic of sharply split states of mind could be considered in the light of the increasingly permissive society developing in the 1960s and early 1970s. What sense could people make of the poor fit between the ideas of retributive justice so often dominating the morality of small children, which could be felt through projective processes as painful pressures by the adults in charge, and the conscious beliefs of these same adults in a softer morality that valued understanding and was reluctant to impose too many limits and penalties? This sort of struggle has to be reworked in every work discussion seminar, and it involves clarifying and critiquing the values of contemporary institutions alongside the study of how individuals create their own meanings.

One of the tricky aspects of work discussion groups is always the realization that the relationship between staff in the work setting will provide some of the points of painful conflict that the seminar member needs to discuss. This is made easier if the seminar is composed of people from entirely different settings and, of course, also underlines the necessity for preliminary discussion of the confidentiality of material presented in the group and exploration of how suitable anonymity of professional colleagues will be maintained. Sometimes people resort to initials to avoid names, but these can feel quite dehumanizing; changes of name are an alternative, though often difficult to adhere to systematically under the pressure of emotional material. There is discussion elsewhere in this book of adaptations of method required when the seminar members are all working in the same place, as in the chapter by Emil Jackson. But discomfort usually accompanies the description of staff conflict, partly because the differential status inherent in adult–child interactions is no longer protective of the individual, and the revelation of personal weaknesses is feared. For example, one teacher doing small-group work in a primary school described her profoundly upset and almost paranoid reaction to a decision by a class teacher to remove one of the members of the small group because of other priorities in the class. She was quite unable to imagine that the child's improved state of mind might make her now an asset in the classroom, believing instead that one of her babies was being stolen from her, and feeling in a panic about her vulnerable position in the school. It was very interesting to link this potential breakdown of adult cooperation to the social context of these children's families, most of whom were very recent immigrants to the United Kingdom, thus having lost the support of the wider extended family and quite often having left children behind in the home country, to be cared for by grandmothers. The worker's identification with a child who could not be properly shared and with a mother figure deprived of a child and in an anxious and distressed state of mind seemed likely to be fuelled by these unconscious associations. The method of work in the seminar allowed these connections to emerge in a manageable way because the idea offered for exploration was that the worker's being upset was likely to be something to do with the meaning for the child of the movement between small group and class that could be thought about.

The contribution of the theory of containment

As Gianna Williams and Beta Copley proposed in an earlier unpublished review of work discussion, the overarching theory of greatest relevance is Bion's theory of containment. This "stepping stone in development" (Bion) proved the flexible idea that could be powerfully employed to support workers and hence the children in their care. The containment offered by the seminar and the tasks of written preparation and conversational exploration set for its members proved to have a usually reliable impact. A new space, which amplified the resources of individuals at work, was created. People's minds grew, and new ideas could be considered because the seminar was felt to be a safe place for confusion, depression, uncertainty, and a sense of being overwhelmed or incompetent to be described, as well as a place to enjoy happier aspects of people's work. The role of the seminar leader is explored in greater detail in chapter 2, but what it required fundamentally was someone who could create a non-judgemental atmosphere, promote curiosity and hopefulness, bear disappointment, relate to the seminar members as creative people, and sustain a culture of equality. Insights offered and carefully grounded in the details of what had been discovered were not so liable to be elevated to *ex cathedra* status and idealized but, instead, to be available as work in progress. Future seminar discussions could review what had proved useful and what would need to be revised.

The seminar leader's function is evidently parental in some respects, and indeed the nature of the task bears comparison with that described as characteristic of "couple family" functioning by Harris and Meltzer in their delineation of forms of family life (Meltzer & Harris, 1986). There have been interesting variations made in work discussion methods in specific contexts, including one well-established within the context of a course for teachers on the emotional aspects of teaching and learning, in which a pair of seminar leaders work with a rather larger group of students: ten, as compared with the normal five or six (Hartland-Rowe, 2005; Youell, 2006). This makes for a sense of a parental couple working together and able to share the more maternal and paternal aspects of the task between them. We might see these broadly and schematically as supportive, nurturing, encouraging, and providing time and space on the one hand, and challenging, limit-setting, stimulating, and exciting on the other. Where there are two leaders, they can engage in dialogue both within, and also subsequent to, seminars, and this models at best the creative conjunction of different perspectives. For a single seminar leader, the process has to be more internal, with the aim being to achieve a balance of receptive support and the challenge of the new—not so very different from the task of psychoanalytic psychotherapists in their clinical work.

Recurrent themes in work discussion

In thinking about the evolution of work discussion, it has been interesting to gather up some of the themes and characteristic directions that emerge from a very wide reading of work discussion papers and seminar material. The later chapters in the book provide many detailed examples but they each have a highly specific context and it may therefore be useful to note here some regularly recurring preoccupations.

Prominent preoccupations in work discussion seminars are the importance of beginnings and endings and the impact of loss and separation. These reflect the experience both of workers and of the children they work with and are relevant to the life histories of many of the troubled children they encounter—loss of parents by death, abandonment, and marital breakdown, loss of country and community through war and exile, and the many less dramatic but searing deprivations arising from disability, maternal depression, poverty, and social exclusion, and, indeed, the ordinary management of transitions, such as that from home to nursery. The opportunity in the work setting for children and adolescents' anxieties linked to separation and loss to be reworked in the relationships formed with significant adults is a discovery made by many. Institutional turbulence is often a spur. Nurseries, schools, inpatient adolescent units, children's homes all experience staff changes, managerial reorganization, and sometimes merger or closure. Even staff illness and absences and the comings and goings of staff rotas can be seen to have a great impact on the security and the state of mind of the children. Acting out becomes more marked, sometimes to a frightening degree when potentially self-harming young people are disturbed by such changes.

In understanding these reactions, there is a richness of theory to draw upon—both the psychoanalytic literature on mourning and depression by Freud, Klein, Winnicott, and others, and the literature from attachment theory developed by Bowlby and current attachment researchers. The clinical work of child psychotherapists over the last three decades with severely deprived children, particularly those in the care system, has helped to make these theoretical ideas accessible to those who work with disturbed children, particularly throwing light on the phenomenon of "double deprivation" (Henry, 1974), when a deprived child becomes identified with a cruelly depriving internal figure and is, in consequence, very difficult to reach or to help through offering a better experience in the here and now.

Play is a vital part of work with children, and learning to be able to think about a child's state of mind through observing play is a central plank of work discussion, often building explicitly on the observation of toddlers and young children, which is a frequent accompanying seminar experience. Finding a position in relation to a child's play or incapacity to play is a complex matter and is, of course, connected to the definition of the worker's role. In nursery work, there is a plethora of possible positions for the adult to take—to supervise group play, to accompany an individual child or small group through the attentiveness of close observation, to lead or organize activity, or to be a "play-partner" (Bruner, Jolly, & Sylva, 1976), following the child's lead.

More difficult and distressing is the encounter with children who cannot play. The pain to which the worker who pauses to watch closely can be exposed is often startling. For example, here is a description of the response to nursery of a boy of 2¼ who spoke almost no English:

> Amir is sitting on the chair by the doors, focusing on the space in front of him with a blank and dull expression in his moist dark brown eyes. His hands are tightly clutching his blue bag. He remained seated on the chair from the time his mother left him at 1 p.m. until the time she came back to pick him up at 3.30 p.m. As I felt very concerned, I asked the nursery nurse about him, and she reassured me in a detached tone of voice that he was "doing OK, actually" and was "becoming much better". Later she sighed and added, "At least, he has stopped screaming—he used to cry all the time. Now he just sits there and does not want to join in."

> Amir continued his practice of waiting for his mother to return while sitting on the same blue chair each day for nearly a whole term.

The observer was herself struggling with the recognition of the unfamiliarity of the complex multicultural mix of the nursery, very much able to identify with this boy's sense of disorientation and panic in her awareness of not understanding the children's mother tongue or knowing much about their cultural background.

The diverse theories of the development of the capacity to play and of impediments to play offered by psychoanalytic theory, developmental researchers, educationalists, and clinicians provide a rich literature to explore.

The opportunity for discovering the complexity and variety of children's lives in the United Kingdom was, for me, a wholly unexpected aspect of the work discussion seminar experience. Class, cultures, religion, regional difference, ethnicity, sexual mores all make themselves felt once details are attended to. One unusual example of this were the reports of a support teacher for Traveller children (Dollery, 2002). She found herself understanding gradually why the early good achievements of Traveller children at school tended to tail off dramatically. Their parents did not really see the sense of education beyond the age of 11—by that age, the community believed, the children could and should be working, and school simply infantilized them. She also observed that whereas schools—and she herself—believed in individual development as the aim of education, Travellers saw the group identity as the important one, and too much focus on an individual as a threat to group cohesion. She puzzled over the concrete thinking the children seemed to continue to display despite their maturing in other ways. Reflecting on this, in an unpublished paper arising from her participation in a work discussion seminar, she wrote:

> It is a community that responds and acts in a very concrete way. There is little space for reflection. The culture not only encompasses physical movement from one place to another but also a continual mental shift away from difficult thoughts and feelings. On many occasions when speaking to the parents, my head becomes cloudy and I find it hard to take things in, as though my thinking capacity is also being interfered with. Negative feelings cannot be held onto and are quickly discharged, often through acts of violence both within the family and wider community.
>
> This cultural inability to take in, reflect upon and digest nega-

> tive experiences results in a lack of containment for the children, leading to difficulties in thinking and symbolising. Melanie Klein's concept of "Epistemophilia" (Klein, M., 1931), the child's wish to learn being linked to curiosity about the mother's body and later her mind, is also severely inhibited. Sexuality is a taboo subject for these children. Bodies are kept covered, babies are universally bottle-fed. Underclothes are washed and hidden under towels. Children are usually refused permission to attend sex education classes.

She also tried to understand the women's inability to do anything about frequent domestic violence: they would depart to a refuge with the children, but then simply return a few days later, with flimsy promises from their husbands. This is how she came to describe the form of cohesion with the Traveller community:

> Those Travellers who do work have jobs that depend on employment from the settled community, making it rather a symbiotic relationship. A definition of gang mentality I came across seems relevant to this. "The gang-family, by virtue of its ambiguous relation to the community, at once defiant and yet seeking acceptance, greedy and at the same time scornfully proud, imposes a confusing task on its members."
>
> My experience is that defences of hostility amongst Travellers are rather brittle and skin deep. Throughout history, there have been periods of extermination of Travelling people. The legacy of this destruction is a lack of an imbued sense of good self-esteem within the culture. Indeed it seems to me that the culture itself serves as a "second skin equivalent", giving Travellers a sense that the rudimentary parts of their personality can somehow be held together, as long as they remain members of the group. In this way, the Travellers on site tend to develop the social appearances of a personality but seem to lack a sense of inner mental space and internal resources.
>
> Existence within the community seems to be one of "adhesive identification" to the basic assumption of the group, namely that threats lie outside.

We can see that work discussion has provided her with theories about group process (basic assumptions, gang mentality) as well as ideas about individual psychic development (the epistemophilic instinct, projection, symbolization, intolerance of mental pain) and that the two forms of theoretical understanding are joined in her interesting suggestion that Traveller culture itself serves as a kind of "second skin" for a fragile and frightened community.[2]

Conclusion

These examples of theoretical resource and theorized discovery, as in the work with the Traveller children, bring us to the question of the place of theory in work discussion seminars. Doubtless there are substantial variations in practice, but an agreed emphasis would be to focus on the material brought to the seminar and the elaboration of its possible meanings in the responses within the group. The mode of learning is not, of course, theory-free—the structure of the seminar and the leader's responses are profoundly rooted in theoretical assumptions, as discussed earlier—but theory is kept in the background. Suggestions about what people might like to read to follow up ideas and insights are likely to include a considerable range: psychoanalytic and child psychotherapy literature, child development texts, the analysis of group and institutional life, social theory, and also works of literature, including children's literature. But the seminars themselves will often include little explicit theoretical discussion, although this generalization has to be set alongside the fact that each particular mix of members and seminar leader produces a unique constellation. This model of education is, I believe, fundamentally transferable and adaptable. The question of how much theory to make available and also the nature and range of the theories that are drawn on is an open one. The psychoanalytic framework described here has proved workable and fertile, but it seems entirely possible that other theoretical perspectives could be combined with the core approach.

It seems appropriate here to summarize briefly my view of the aims and methods of the work discussion groups as they have evolved. Let us imagine a particular seminar early in the life of a group's existence. It starts with clarification of the worker's role and tries to describe as fully as possible what is happening in the interactions reported, to discuss what the child is conveying, and to take account of what is evoked for the worker while safeguarding the worker's own privacy. There is no expectation of finding an answer, but a commitment to facilitating thinking. To do this, the individuals and the group between them need to hold things in mind, to learn to listen, to appreciate the containing potential of setting and institution, to think about what might be helpful (and be realistic about what help is available and appropriate in the setting), to learn to hear and also to use different forms of communication, and to consider others' perceptions of the situation. Attention to boundaries of time and place and to issues of confidentiality are background commitments, as is the struggle to be in touch with the feelings, conscious and unconscious, of everyone involved. What this means in practice for the development of sensitivity and the expansion of skills and understanding is what the rest of this book is about.

Notes

1. This methodology was also adapted for use with physiotherapists by Stanford Bourne and reported in Bourne (1981), *Under the Doctor: Studies in the Psychological Problems of Physiotherapists, Patients and Doctors*.

2. This understanding, obtained from work discussion of the psychosocial dynamics of a Traveller community, provides a vivid illustration of Mary Douglas's "grid-group" analysis of social forms. This community seems like an enclave, in Douglas's four-fold typology, giving its dominant priority to the preservation of group identity over individual opportunities (see Douglas, 1970).

CHAPTER TWO

The work discussion seminar: a learning environment

Jonathan Bradley

This chapter considers the potential for and process of learning in a work discussion seminar. The relationship between the seminar leader and the members of the group is at the heart of the learning experience. The material brought to the seminar is often profoundly painful and upsetting for both presenter and listeners. The crucial role of the seminar leader is in finding a way for the group to become aware of the nature of the distress being communicated by the worker, and by client to worker, to be able to hold on to it for long enough to get beyond immediate defensive responses, and ultimately to understand more about how the worker's relationship to the client may be able to modulate the emotional situation helpfully.

This kind of learning becomes possible as the seminar leader directs members' attention away from learning additional facts and towards reflection on practice. Those taking part in a seminar may well find that no one else there shares their profession. This could lead to a view of their being the undisputed expert in their field or, by contrast, allow them to become part of a group where they are free to reflect on their work in a different way. The seminar leader's task is to help the group to move in this direction.

A process of learning that boldly asserts that there will be no explicit teaching of techniques puzzles people at first but becomes fascinating as the method gathers steam. On the whole, the written description of work brought to the seminar is sufficient for the task of the group, though interesting additional details are sometimes remembered during the discussion. The process can at first be quite disturbing, as new questions start to arise within areas of work in which the worker had felt quite competent. At times the group can feel that it is being invited to participate in a process of "unlearning" rather than of learning. There is initially a delicate balance between a focus on the material presented and the contributions by others present, including the seminar leader. The task of the group as a whole is to be supportive of a process that will involve a fresh consideration of what may have been hitherto held rather unquestioningly. The seminar leader has to combine encouraging the study of the personality interactions described and the exploration of the influence of unconscious processes with an awareness of any defensive obstructive processes that may be aroused in the group.

Insights gained about unconscious dynamics go beyond the particular presentation and its subject matter and allow members to have a memorable learning experience that can be applied to many other situations. It is moving to witness a moment when insight is gained by the group as a whole. But this is not the only possibility: sometimes one or two members will stand out in terms of their capacity for insight; at other times a member will be left behind and struggle emotionally, leading to a feeling of anxiety in the group as a whole. And, of course, there can be a move against new learning in the whole group, which the seminar leader has to deal with.

I will illustrate some of these themes by describing two work discussion presentations in some detail.

Case 1: dealing with renal failure

A member of the group, a paediatric nurse, presented an account of Juliette, a teenager who had to deal with the terrible consequences of a late diagnosis of meningitis. Not only did she suffer from chronic renal failure, but due to the way the blood supply was withdrawn by the body system, she had to have both legs amputated at the knee, lost finger tips on one hand, and all the fingers except her thumb on the other hand. She had had skin grafts taken from her abdomen and had also had surgery to help her pass stools and urine. Despite this, she was able to go to school and was working hard to catch up with her GCSEs.

I need hardly describe what a profound effect this account had on the work discussion group. There was a sense of incredulity that any teenager's life could have been turned upside down so tragically. As a group—and I include myself—we struggled to be informed about renal failure, learning about the various techniques that are employed to provide kidney function. This search for information provided an opportunity for the group to become "ordinary learners" at a very stressful time, when it was very difficult to put oneself in the place of the tragic young girl presented. But this process of educating ourselves was not powerful enough to contain all our feelings. For example, mention was made of one consequence of dialysis: namely, that very little liquid is allowed to the patient. In fact, patients have to become accustomed to feeling "parched" all the time, and they often have severe headaches as the body protests against such a strict regime. Though there was, of course, a world of difference between this account, delivered in a seminar, and the impact of being on a renal ward, nevertheless there was a powerful communication of what it would feel like to have one's water supply restricted in this way. The response was somatic rather than reflective. Small water bottles brought into the seminar for refreshment (the equivalent of a day's supply for a renal patient) were sought for in bags and felt for reassurance, and there were several journeys to the toilet. Out of the blue, a primitive way of dealing with a painful situation thus took centre stage, the somatic response being the price to be paid for the group's struggle to respond in an attentive and emotionally present way to this painful scenario. I remember, as seminar leader, feeling enormous concern for them and wondering whether they were being asked to cope with too much. Events proved that I was being over-anxious on their behalf since, after a brief drinks interlude, there was a determined return to task.

The following is an account of an evening on evening/night duty with Juliette. The presenter established, when coming on duty, that Juliette had asked if the nurse could watch videos with her during the evening before another serious operation. A number of duties with other patients had to be carried out before she could go to Juliette.

> Juliette got up and we went to the cupboard. I asked her what type of movies she liked. She shrugged in answer. So I randomly picked video titles and suggested them to her for her selection. After a few suggestions, Juliette asked me what I wanted to watch. I told her that as long as it was not scary, I would watch it with her. We finally picked about five videos and returned to her room.

Juliette chose the Rugrats to watch, and I put that in. She took her prosthetic legs off and scratched her right leg where there was a dressing. I asked her if she was OK, and she said she was fine. We watched about 20 minutes, and then Juliette decided it was boring, so I changed it to a video of the Chipmunks.

Juliette asked if she could have some fruit squash instead of plain water. She was having gut surgery, which required that she was not to have food for 24 hours and have clear fluids till 10.30 on the morning of surgery. So I double-checked with the nurse in charge and got her a cup of orange squash. In the time it took me to do that, she had decided that this movie was also boring. So we changed the video to Andre. We watched a few minutes of it, and the door buzzed. . . .

I returned to Juliette, who had put her supra-pubic catheter on free drainage as her normal routine. She was scratching her arms and abdomen. I asked if she was OK, and she said she was a little itchy. I suggested that it was time to take her medication, but she preferred to take them a little later. So we watched the movie. Then she began a conversation.

J[uliette]: Is it going to hurt, what they'll do tomorrow?

N[urse]: I don't know much about the surgery but since it's on your abdomen, I think it will hurt some. But I'm sure you'll get some pain relief.

J: What is morphine?

N: It is a pain relief medicine which we can give in your mouth or via a cannula, and you can push a button when you're in pain and receive a dose. It's called a PCA, which you control.

J: What about going after?

N: Do you mean when you pass stool?

J: Yes.

N: Well, it's going to be a while before you do that, but I don't know.

J: But what do you think?

N: Well, I think it shouldn't hurt, because I don't think they are going to touch anything in that area. I think it's only going to be your stomach they touch.

J: When can I eat?

N: I think possibly the day after your surgery.

J: What! I would have been starved for two days. That's not happening. I'll eat. I don't care what anyone says.

[*At this moment I thought I should back-track and reassure her, since I was guessing.*]

N: Well they are going to handle your bowel, which is part of your gut, and this will affect when you can eat.

J: But this is about pooing, not eating.

N: Well, it's all linked from your mouth right to your anus.

J: You know that it is a mile long. A mile long, all in there.

[*She pointed to her stomach.*]

N: You are right about that. How come the person who "consented" you did not speak to you about the procedure?

J: The doctor who came was rude and nasty.

N: That's not fair on you. Listen, I'll say at handover that the surgeon needs to speak to you before the procedure so that you can ask your questions. And one of us can be with you if it helps.

J: OK.

Juliette asked me to get her lucky pyjamas. I did, and then asked her to take her medication, as her scratching had become more frantic. She sat up and put about eight tablets into her mouth at once, took a drink, and swallowed them all.

Discussion

The account is a moving blend of questions that are harrowing in their simplicity and a routine intended to reassure and allow difficult procedures to take place. Many details about hospital life emerged in discussion. Some procedures had to be carried out by the surgeons, and this would involve sending a patient away from the ward. What place would there be for adolescent anxieties such as where a scar would be left due to the passing of blood through the dialysis machine? Would it be below the neckline or above the elbow, so that it could be hidden? What to make of the possibly divergent opinions between medical staff, the teenagers, and their parents? Would it be dangerous to acknowledge that this could be an important issue to discuss, given the life-and-death quality of the work on the ward? For example, a site on the arm below the elbow was often chosen for the link to the dialysis machine when operating, so that if it became infected, it would still be possible to insert another above the elbow. The price of failure would be savage.

It seemed possible that these simple yet heartbreaking questions were being evaded, since the consequences of trying to give an answer would uncover other questions for Juliette, such as "How on earth did I lose limbs, continence, the possibility of a sexual life because of a delay in correctly diagnosing a headache?" Enormous efforts were being made to keep Juliette alive and motivated to live. There seemed to be a very fragile line between supporting her efforts to emerge from a state of withdrawal from life and allowing her to voice something of her pain and rage at what had happened, with all its dreadful consequences.

It was clear to me that there was enormous tension in the seminar room at times. The group was distressed at being part of a life-and-death drama played out behind a scene characterized by a succession of trivia. How could the facts of bilateral amputation, the loss of fingers, the insertion of catheters, and anxiety about the imminent operation be reconciled with the picture of the dedicated schoolgirl hoping to achieve good marks at GCSE, or with the apparently insignificant request for orange squash rather than plain water? It seemed gradually to become clear that while the members of the group were following the banality of the conversation, they felt filled close to bursting point with the intensity of the tragedy. There was a sense of being asked to bear something apparently missing from the day-to-day exchanges on the ward. Why was there such a disparity between the acutely painful circumstances of the patient and the muted reactions of hospital staff who were dealing in such a matter-of-fact way with this tragic situation? A similar imbalance seemed to be observable within the seminar itself, particularly in the interchange between the presenter and the rest of the group. Dialogue was difficult for a while, and it seemed that the presenter felt she had to defend the good reputation of the hospital and hold on to a rigid definition of her job.

My dilemma was that while I was aware of the impatience—even desperation—of the seminar group for something interpretative to be said to Juliette, I felt great sympathy for the plight of her nurse, who was clearly troubled by not feeling able to expand her role. In fact, I was strongly put in mind of a similar situation I had encountered when carrying out some consultancy work with nurses from a hospital ward on which there were a number of very sick children, many of whom did not recover. I was grateful for the way in which this situation came to my mind when I felt quite caught between opposing views and could see no clear way of taking the discussion forward. I will describe what I found myself recalling.

> My consultation had been arranged by the medical consultant who felt that the nurses would be helped by having a regular space to talk and think about the harrowing situations they had to deal with. I was very impressed by the quality of the work being carried out, but, from the beginning, it was apparent that there was a feeling of ambivalence in the group. The group could manage neither to attend regularly nor to describe their work when asked to do so. The presentations were usually verbal, and it was stated by a number of presenters that they had not felt able to sit and write down what had happened. They felt that what happened on the ward was dire enough, but to write something down would be to invite unwanted feelings to return, whereas all they wanted to do was to forget them.
>
> This was illustrated powerfully by one nurse describing a disturbing time spent with a girl of just 4 years, suffering from the effects of an aggressive cancer. As she sat with her, she found herself hoping that the girl would die. The medical staff seemed to have a different viewpoint. Indeed, the girl's deteriorating condition was pushing them to further action, as they obtained the parents' permission to administer a newly developed drug in the hope that it would lead to a halt in the inexorable progress of the cancer. The intervention was not successful, and the little girl died at 3 o'clock in the morning. The nurse presenting was clearly very upset at her feelings at that time. She went on to say that it was Christmas morning, and she was on duty three hours later. Indeed, some time previously she had volunteered to be Father Christmas, and found herself forcing "Ho, Ho, Ho's" out of her mouth while the rest of her was "in the same place as the little girl" (her words). In other words, feeling that life had ended. Later that day, to her surprise and subsequent embarrassment, she became extremely irritated with the parent of another child who had complained to her that one of the hospital's TV sets had very poor reception, and this was ruining their favourite programme. She was so angry with them about what she regarded as selfishness that she could barely wait till the end of her shift, when she was able to do "kick-boxing" to get it out of her system.

> When she had finished her account, most of the group nodded their assent. They clearly expected me to dispute the premise that events that are very upsetting need to be got rid of rather than be processed. I felt challenged to defend the decision to convene a meeting about their work, and I felt that unless the defence of it came from within the group itself, this would be the end. At that moment, in the mind of the group, I seemed to be experienced as an "annoying" parent who came with nagging requests while they were trying to deal with great tragedy. The group managed to say that these meetings could not possibly mean as much to me as to them. To me, they said, it was a job, however sympathetically it was carried out. They, on the other hand, had to cope with death on a daily basis. They had no space for reflection: they just had to get on with their job, ready for the next death. It was powerfully said. To my relief, one of the nurses offered a different view. She said that she was very grateful for the nurse's account. She had not known what a particularly difficult Christmas Day she had had. Her words had moved her very much and had helped her to recall the child, with whom she also had spent time. It made her sad, but she felt it was better to remember rather than just forget the pain. She felt privileged to be with the children. They were special people, and being with them helped her as a person.
>
> Her words, deeply felt, moved the whole group. Afterwards, I found myself wondering about the different responses to the presentation, one to defend against emotional suffering and the other embracing it as a necessary price for keeping in touch with what mattered, without which one risked being cut off from one's own feelings.

This digression will, I hope, have served to illustrate the situation I encountered in the seminar while considering the material from the renal unit. The presenter's position was a complex one. One concern was how to manage the routine of death on the ward, and at the same time how to help patients to go on with their lives, no matter how catastrophic their illness and injuries. As a consequence, a patient's merest indication of a wish to have a future tended to be seized upon. A particular anxiety was that there should be no visible sign of an operation having taken place. Hence the pressure on nurses to be able to promise that once they had left hospital, patients would be able to wear a "bikini" without visible scars. Parents sometimes arranged for skin graft operations to take place in addition to the extensive operations that had already taken place, often over many years. It was as if the unrealistic hope of a body without blemish, the restoration of a "perfect daughter", was a way of holding on to the hope that not everything had been hopelessly damaged. Perhaps the "bikini" test was deliberately extreme in order to combat the impact of an illness, which took away the dignity of being able to carry out basic bodily functions and which required particularly intrusive medical interventions. The presenter felt under immense pressure to go along with the culture of the ward, even though she had severe misgivings about it.

But what of the response of the seminar group to this scenario? There was a powerful realization within the group that they were in fact in touch with a quite appropriate sense of sadness and despair—feelings that could not be voiced easily by Juliette or the nurses on the ward. It was at this point that terms I had mentioned in discussion, such as "evacuation" "projection" and "splitting", took on a very different meaning. The group had experienced something emotionally profound. They were able to apply psychoanalytic concepts to their understanding in an experiential way. It was quite clear that learning in this way was quite different from merely learning about something, as if it were merely a descriptive process.

The group's realization of the major forces set loose by such tragedies made it possible for horizons to be broadened and other issues to be considered. It was possible, for example, to consider some larger institutional issues. Did counselling on the ward have to be considered only as a formal referral option, or would it be possible to think about the emotional needs of patients in a less formal way and in an everyday context? This question led to thoughtful discussion about what sort of comment might be made to a child on the ward, and to a greater understanding of the importance of ongoing relationships within the ward setting. Ultimately, the presenter herself felt sufficiently supported by the seminar setting to raise the following broad questions about practice:

- Why does looking after a sick child make it difficult to look beyond the physical needs?
- Why is it difficult to organize a team, communicate effectively, and listen?
- How does one help a child to understand their own mortality?
- Are the boundaries of a nurse's role the real obstacle to allow-

ing some thinking/talking beyond the physical problems requiring care?

- Is it lack of time or fear of what might be said or revealed that makes it difficult to start talking about the emotional and psychological issues?

These questions were related to some further reflective points explored in the seminar:

- the effect of working in a high-stress, high-demand environment
- dealing with life and death every day
- the difficulty of providing real emotional support, to allow space for patients and parents
- a setting very focused on the pathophysiology issues, with comparatively little time invested in the psychological or emotional side of the patients' care.
- lack of resources outside the hospital for the continued provision of support once the patient has been discharged.

It will be evident how wide-ranging are the issues the seminar members could gradually struggle with in response to this particular presentation.

Case 2: reflecting on loss

The previous case presentation concerned a situation within which the worker had to expand her usual practice to introduce flexibility to a narrowly defined job description. My experience is that this is a characteristic outcome over time for many members of work discussion groups. However, I now want to refer to a different kind of problem: one in which the worker also had a well-defined role within a well-established therapeutic community. The main issue did not centre on the definition of work, but on whether and how contact could be made with an emotionally vulnerable boy.

Ryan was referred to the community at the age of 6½ years. It was clear from case notes that by the time he reached the community, he had had 17 residential placement changes in his first two years, and 40 altogether. He had been subjected to much abuse and had witnessed extreme domestic violence. He was prone to explosive bouts of rage, and this had probably played an active part in the breakdown of a number of his placements. An extremely challenging aspect of Ryan's behaviour was his soiling, which seemed to be constant. He would soil his pants and avoid the use of toilets, finding "special" places for depositing his faeces. He was always on the edge of the group, avoiding company where possible, and the smell of his incontinence ensured the effectiveness of his avoidance strategy.

Alongside this behaviour, the ordered regularity of life in the community began to make its presence felt. This was nothing dramatic, but for the first time in Ryan's life there was a regime of clear and consistent boundaries, intended to convey a sense of proportion, predictability, and reliability. Workers were encouraged to value the significance of paying attention to the fine details of every child's living experience. Even so, it was not until Ryan had been at the community for a year that he seems to have begun to entertain the tentative hope that his stay—already the longest period he had spent in any one place—might go on for some time. He began to make tentative moves in the direction of his male keyworker, who was a member of a work discussion seminar. Intuitively he had chosen the person who had been on the staff group for the longest time. Over the next year, the beginnings of a relationship began to take shape. Painfully, as the expectation of regularity began to take root, so too did a greater awareness of any absence. The community tried to be sensitive to this by introducing the concept of a worker couple, whereby Mary, another worker in the home, would cover the absences of Ryan's keyworker. In the seminar, we discussed how this arrangement mirrored the case of a parental couple. The following is an account of his reaction to this initiative, at a time when there was also an attempt being made to think with him about his past placements through "life-story work":

> Ryan burst out of the room where we were working and had been talking about how Mary would look after him when I was not there, and retreated in a noisy commotion to his bedroom. When I followed him, he jumped up from his bed in an angry rage. Still clutching Whitey (a pet sheep) in his hand, he then proceeded to kick his toy box across the room. The contents exploded onto the floor, producing chaos in his room. With a shrill voice he began to swear at me, repeatedly calling me a "Bitch" and saying that he hated me. Ryan picked up a heavy toy car and threw it at me but narrowly missed, and it hit the wall. I decided at this

point to stop Ryan, with the aim of at least physically containing some of these powerful feelings. . . . I held him, sitting on the floor just outside his room, away from the chaos. His emotional state quickly changed from anger to noisy excitability, shrieking over any words of reassurance I was trying to offer. At this point Mary came up to support me, having heard the commotion. Ryan almost immediately launched a verbal attack on Mary, swearing and saying that he hated her. His aggression increased again, and he was now kicking out in the direction of Mary. I commented at this point that it seemed that recently he had been taking a lot of his angry feelings out on Mary.

A short while later I returned to the subject, once Ryan appeared a bit calmer. I told him that Mary and I had noticed that when I'm away from the community, there is often an increase in Ryan finding things difficult and that, almost without fail, he seems to take out his difficult feelings on Mary. I then added that it was my experience that often when I am around, Ryan pretends that everything is fine and that I see very little difficult behaviour. Ryan at this point became annoyed and denied this. I asked him how he felt about me having the next two days off. Ryan looked cross but didn't answer. He attempted instead to change the subject and, interestingly, began to talk about his wobbly tooth. Ryan said, "I'm going to pull out my tooth, and when I do, blood is going to go everywhere!" At this point I reassured him that it was very natural for teeth to come out (thinking to myself that this was a wonderful image of a necessary separation) and that even though it was a bit worrying and maybe painful, things normally turned out OK.

Comment

On listening to this account, I was impressed by two very different targets of Ryan's rage. The first was the launching of objects into an unboundaried space, with no way of knowing or being able to control the effects of what is launched. The heavy toy car carried murderous intent with it. The second episode certainly describes furious rage, but here, the worker's own body marks the boundary, as does his thinking presence. A boy who for a long time could only skulk at the periphery of things was able to launch an attack and come to realize that it could be contained, that he would not inevitably destroy his carer, as had happened so many times before when his placement had broken down as a consequence of his violent behaviour. I was put very much in mind of Bion's comment that if, as Melanie Klein states, an excessive amount of projective identification is harmful, then we can assume that a certain amount is necessary. In this case the experience of having to cope with the absence of his keyworker could only be described as the equivalent of an empty cavity, of nothing being there for Ryan, and he is preoccupied with broadcasting the damage that he feels has been done to him. Nevertheless, after some years in the community, a fuller picture is emerging than that presented by his avoidant and incontinent behaviour, which had as its main aim the disguise of his anxious hopes of containment.

The seminar group were very moved by the courage shown by this boy as he began to emerge from his state of angry withdrawal. They felt deeply involved in supporting the work of the keyworker, who was able to continue to think creatively while under enormous pressure. At times, being the recipient of Ryan's pained reaction to loss was almost too much to bear. There was one occasion, for example, when after a number of years in the community Ryan was on the point of leaving a successful weekend camp at which he had been staying with other looked-after children. At the moment of departure he broke down and cried for 40 minutes. Eventually *"he wiped his eyes and said that he didn't ever want to say goodbye to any more people. He then began to describe a pain in his stomach, which felt empty and sore."* To the worker, as well as being painful to bear, this moment felt like a great development: Ryan was able to put into words his feelings about loss and separation and also, movingly, about his sense of attachment.

Conclusion: a matter of chemistry

I would like to conclude this chapter by commenting on what has emerged about the setting of the work discussion seminar, and particularly about the relationship between the seminar group and the seminar leader. The setting is, of course, very important, since it provides a foundation upon which learning can take place. The fundamentals of the setting become reliably familiar: regular meetings over a two-year period; equal opportunity among the group for presentation of work on a predictable basis; the opportunity to look closely at interactions; the emergence of insight into the situation discussed. These are, of course, also fundamental elements of the clinical psychoanalytic setting. But in the case of work discussion other quite different elements are present as well. The seminar leader needs to be active in creating a non-judgemental atmosphere, in promoting curiosity, sustaining the group at times of despair, and treating group members with respect. At first sight these two aims, the analytic and the developmental, seem at loggerheads with each other, the one essentially passive and the other active. In fact, they are complementary. Some time ago, when writing about supervision (Bradley, 1997), I described the main challenge of supervision as that of providing useful insights into the relationship between therapist and patient, which, by its very nature, is private and exclusive. The most important role of the supervisor, in my view, is to facilitate communication between therapist and patient and to augment the resources available for dealing with crises within the treatment rather than attempt to take over command, and conduct the therapy at one remove. In many ways, the role of the seminar leader is similar. One is there to allow a process to take place, not to take it over. The promoting of curiosity is therefore a complex aim and might be viewed as a double-edged sword. The seminar leader can help to promote learning in the group but can, if too insistent, also stifle the group's own wish to learn. One needs to hold on to the expectation that if the group remain focused, a clearer understanding will emerge. Memorably, Bion (quoted in Harris, 1987) describes the meeting between analyst and analysand as giving rise to disturbance, which he called an "emotional storm". He says that throughout the process "storm-tossed but not shaken", the analyst must go on thinking clearly. This more disciplined reaction builds up strength and courage and a capacity to stand fast. Bion assumes that very often the analyst will not realize consciously what is happening, but, he says, "if we stay, do not run away . . . go on observing the patient, after a time a pattern will emerge" (quoted in Harris, 1987, p. 342).

I think there are parallels here with many situations brought to work discussion seminars. They may have been deeply distressing or frustrating to the worker, and the feelings aroused may be accompanied by an inability to think about what is going on. This was certainly true of the hospital episode described earlier. The group immersed itself emotionally in the world of the patient and the nurse and was encouraged to do so by me, rather than taking up a more intellectual enquiry into the hospital situation and thus making suggestions about practice without fully appreciating the enormous difficulty of being open to the emotional impact of hospital life. The thoughts that eventually emerged seemed to me to be rooted in an understanding of complexity and, as such, could be transforming of hospital practice, if developed and sustained.

In many ways I felt, as a seminar leader, that the situation with Ryan was even more difficult to deal with. The facts described were so painful. The group had to think about a young boy who should not have had 40 placement changes before he was 6 years old. Anger and frustration at a social care system that could allow such a sequence of events to take place are easily available as ways of not becoming emotionally involved in the current reality. For, inevitably, the painful issues of separation and loss remind members of their own experience. Money-Kyrle (1956), talking about the analytic situation, describes the patient as standing for those areas within the analyst's own unconscious that are still endangered by aggression and still in need of care and reparation: A partial motive in being concerned for "the patient's well-being is that the patient is the representative of a former immature or ill part of himself, including his damaged objects, which he can now understand and therefore treat by interpretation in the external world" (p. 332).

Money-Kyrle is, of course, speaking of an analytic situation, which the work discussion seminar is not. Nevertheless, I believe that the inevitable frustration with the limitations of one's own work situation does enable students, with the help of a supportive group and seminar leader, to embark on a process of learning that is personally fulfilling. It is, of course, a process that takes time, and I would like to make a final point about the function of time and space, both in relation to the examples discussed in this chapter and in the functioning of the work discussion group. It was noticeable that it was only after a year that Ryan began to entertain the possibility that his stay at the unit might go on for some time. It was at this point that he was able to set up contact with a keyworker and embark tentatively on a relationship, however stormy it was. Such a process requires time (Canham, 1999) and a process within which the earlier abuses of those early years could be challenged by the provision of a thoroughly dependable space, over time, characterized by its sequence of beginnings, moments of contact, and endings. Although this process is most clearly defined by the situation of Ryan, the need for time and space was also present in the situation of Juliette, though in her case there was no time to prepare for a cruel transformation of her life situation. It was the brutal nature of the transformation, giving little space for thought, that was felt so acutely by the work discussion group. The provision of time and space within the seminar setting and the dependability of it formed a very important element in the emergence of thinking linked to emotional experience.

What can be possible in such a setting was well articulated by a student nearing the end of work discussion seminars:

> "I find it easy to substantiate the value of my experience of work discussion on a number of practical levels. Yet of greatest significance to me is the contribution work discussion has made to my own personal development and learning. The value I have gained from the insight and support I have received throughout the seminars has been far-reaching—certainly way beyond my expectations. Indeed, on a daily basis I am reminded of the contribution work discussion has made to my whole life learning, which I am very grateful for."

CHAPTER THREE

What's happening? Some thoughts on the experience of being in a work discussion group

Katie Argent

Going back

Arriving at my first work discussion seminar, I had some idea, gleaned eagerly and anxiously from conversations with other students, about this seminar being to do with conscious and unconscious communication in work with children or young people. I was aware of feeling relieved that as a consequence of my own hard-won experience as a patient in psychoanalytic psychotherapy, I thought I knew a thing or two about unconscious processes that I could now put to good use in what I comfortably imagined would be a fairly abstract though not, of course, impersonal discussion. In other words, I did not arrive with the expectation that this would be a seminar that would touch me emotionally, let alone play a part in changing my perspective on and approach to working life.

As we introduced ourselves in the seminar group, the first surprise was what varied working backgrounds we came from, with widely differing kinds of experience and levels of expertise in work with children and families in areas such as education, health, mental health, social services, and community development. I quickly realized that the array of notepads and pens with which I had armoured myself would not be particularly useful. Rather than studiously taking down references and making notes, we were going to be looking in detail at each other's descriptions of interactions with children and other members of staff in our workplaces, including descriptions of the way in which we ourselves behaved and expressed ourselves in these interactions. Not safely theoretical, then.

And to my further surprise, these descriptions were not meant to aim for objectivity. It took a while and many seminars for it to sink in for me, despite the patient clarity of the seminar leader, that the descriptive task was to grasp the nettle of subjectivity and pay attention to our own thoughts and feelings in the process of observing ourselves in interaction with others at work. In fact what was to be noted, in our minds if not on paper, was what we observed in the widest sense: not only what could be perceived with our eyes and ears, but also the shifts and changes in our own emotional states in order to try to understand the emotional meaning of what we observed. In this, the work discussion seminar called on and sought to develop similar skills and capacities to the baby observation seminar that most of us were doing in parallel. In other ways it was quite distinct, and I explore its distinctiveness from a student's perspective later in this chapter.

Although I had come to the seminar thinking that I was taking a step towards something new, with all the excitement that an idea of fresh starts, clean slates, and brave new worlds can generate, it gradually dawned on me that the kind of work we were doing was more about a revisiting of our working experiences and a re-examining of our prior knowledge and understanding. No blinding flashes of illumination: rather, an opportunity to look again. In this context, after nearly falling off my chair when I met the work discussion seminar leader and recognized her as someone who, many years ago, had been my schoolteacher, I came to think that my sudden sense of going back to school was apt.

Adverbs and adjectives

When the work discussion seminar started, I was working as a teaching assistant in a primary school, based in two Year 2 classes. I presented quite early on in the seminar and proudly brought a carefully recorded account of a series of verbal interactions involving the class teacher, children, and myself, set out in the main as a scripted dialogue. I thought that this would be an accurate and efficient way of presenting what had happened. It went something like this:

Mr W: Do you know why I sent you out?

John: Yes, Mr W.

Mr W: Partly I'm not feeling well, but mostly it was to do with you. Did you have to say something?

John: No, Mr W.

Mr W: Did you feel you just had to say something?

[*Pause*]

John: No, Mr W.

Mr W: Is there something you want to say?

John: Sorry, Mr W.

Mr W: I should hope so. You can go out to play now.

[*John goes out.*]

Mr W [*to me*]: I feel sorry about sending John out, he knows exactly how to wind me up, he doesn't give up.

As we discussed the series of exchanges, I began to see that while what was said was important, a great deal had been missed out in terms of the detail of tone of voice, movement, gesture, and facial expression, let alone the quality of a silence or a stare. What had drawn me to the course of which the seminar was a key part was an interest in finding out more about non-verbal or pre-verbal communication, but this was precisely the area that it seemed difficult to step into when writing up. I could see that I was not alone in finding writing up a challenge and found it puzzling that using lots of adverbs and adjectives, as the seminar leader encouraged us to do and as many of us in the seminar group had had plenty of practice doing in our working lives, appeared now to be a tall order.

There was also the thorny matter of remembering what had happened in order to write it up. Was there a trick to this? Was there perhaps a special knack into which new students would be inducted eventually? How could we be sure that the sequence we thought we remembered was really correct? What if we forgot the essential detail that would make sense of everything else? And then there were the mathematical questions about how much we should be writing and how long this should take us: if it takes half a day to write up one hour's worth of work at 500 words an hour, how many ink cartridges will the average work discussion student need annually for two seminar presentations a term?

Altogether, it became clear that writing up and presenting in seminars could feel uncomfortably exposing, especially to begin with. The benign, facilitating attitude of the seminar leader did much to mediate the sharp end of persecutory anxiety, but I think that embarking on this kind of relatively public looking at oneself in one's working role does tend to stir up strong worries about being seen and judged in a critical light. Trying to remember every single detail, spending hours and hours writing up, or, alternatively, dashing off something in a perfunctory way could all be attempts to manage the discomfort of putting down in writing and presenting to the seminar group our own view of ourselves in relation to others at work. Perhaps becoming preoccupied with these writing-up issues also served to defend against a different kind of exposure: that is, exposure to the impact of complex and sometimes painful emotional states met with in the children and families with whom we worked as well as in ourselves—emotional states that all the adverbs and adjectives were helping to delineate.

Along with the descriptive words, we were starting to learn about what might lie behind an individual style of walking, a vocal pitch, or an atmosphere in a room; about the language of unconscious anxiety, desire, and conflict. We were finding out that what we forgot to write down, what we found ourselves especially struck by, or something—a mood, a manner—that defeated our attempts to put it into words might be valuable indicators in trying to understand what was happening at an emotional level.

What's happening?

Often, when this question was raised following a presentation, we could see that the description showed that something had happened in the class, or student group, or family meeting, or whatever the setting for the presentation was, but not necessarily only at the level of action or conscious communication. The "what's happening?" question invited us to draw out the threads of the presenter's subjective experience, moving in close to focus on the detail, moving out to see the overall shape of the description, bearing in mind the institutional context, organizational dynamics, and the presenter's professional role. When I presented a description of the beginning of a Year 2 school day, the first day of the Year 2 Standard Attainment Tests, thinking with the seminar group about what might be going on at many levels—inter- and intra-personally and organizationally—helped me to understand why the teacher, the children, and I had been so stirred up:

> Mr W catches my eye and grimaces. Sam arrives with his mother and suddenly clings to her with his arms fast around her waist. He buries his head in her jumper. Bemused, she disentangles herself gently. He gestures towards the tables, where sharp pencils and test papers are set out already. Mr W asks him to come and sit down and discourages the other children from lingering around the tables. One of the mothers notices the test papers, and the parents start to pass the news around in loud whispers. Mr W is now extremely calm and authoritative as he ushers parents out and children in. When they are assembled on the carpet, about a quarter of the class seem to be absent. John is talking to his neighbour, and Mr W asks him exasperatedly to stand up. He asks him if he will be able to be quiet, because if not, he will have to leave the room. John stares back with a set jaw and then mumbles defiantly, "Don't know." Mr W shouts at him to go and sit at a distant table. John shuffles over to the table and flops onto a chair. Mr W looks flushed and tired. . . . The children go to sit at their places. Mike moves his chair to be closer to his neighbour and has to be told to move away again. He looks terrified. Lynne lays her head on the table in front of her.

The "what's happening" question also required each of us in the seminar group to consider our own emotional response to what was presented and to try to separate out whatever belonged to our own personal preoccupations from whatever was being communicated by the child, or classroom group, or presenter in the write-up. This could be quite an unsettling process, as dearly held assumptions and beliefs were frequently thrown into question. In presenting work with two individual children in two parallel Year 4 classes, I realized that I was well disposed towards one teacher, who in my descriptions represented a sympathetic, liberal attitude to children, while hostile towards the other teacher, whom I represented as overly strict and firm:

> Ms P sharply tells the class to be quiet. She asks who was doing lines at lunchtime. Four boys put their hands up. I find myself about to put my own hand up. She exasperatedly tells two of

> them to put their hands down because they were not given lines. She holds out her hand for the lines from the remaining two boys and brusquely slaps the paper she is given down on her desk. On the blackboard at the front of the classroom, underneath a detention list, is written "'I must not forget my homework'—write out 25 times." Looking at it, I am aware of feeling sick with fear and fury.

The seminar leader and group wondered about this rather blatant split between nice/good/gentle and horrid/bad/strict teacher as promoted by my descriptions. As I grew more able to disentangle my own anxiety in the strict teacher's classroom from what the child I was working with showed me, I could see that the child himself was thriving within the clear and uncompromising structure provided by the teacher. This was not to say that the strict teacher suddenly acquired a halo: rather, that the seminar helped us to focus on the quality of relationship rather than rushing to make judgements; to look at how an experience was being used rather than categorizing the protagonists as good or bad. In this instance, the experience of being taught by a strict teacher, even an unusually strict teacher, seemed to help the child to find the reliable stability that he needed in order to learn:

> Back in the classroom, Hafid is at first silent when Ms P asks him what he has been doing. She speaks abruptly. Then he tells her in detail about the book he has been reading to me. Watching them talk, I notice that she is focusing on what he is saying with a great deal of warmth and that he is enthusiastic and confident in his response. I suddenly realize that she likes him very much, and he clearly adores her. She asks him seriously if he concentrated on his work or if he went off all over the place. He tells her, smiling, that "we talked". She says firmly that he mustn't.

Sometimes the "what's happening?" had to remain a question for a long time before the presenter and seminar group could start to make sense of what was observed. The process of describing in writing experiences that left us uncertain or uncomprehending and then reflecting on these states of mind and experiences with the seminar leader and group helped with tolerating the frustration of not understanding what we observed and with not leaping prematurely to explanations.

I think that this business of learning to observe ourselves in interaction with others at work and putting this into writing lends itself to a personal investigation of professional role and practice. For some of us, personal psychotherapy helps to support and further this kind of exploration.

Role and responsibility

Having to look at our own role in and contribution to what happens at work can be thought-provoking and energizing; it can also be demanding and difficult. This kind of observation is bound to draw attention to the scope and limitations of professional role, and one's own capacity to address these. In my seminar group serious questions about role and responsibility were raised for each of us. Was participating in this seminar a discrete activity, separate from our actual working lives, or was part of the seminar's function to enable us to take what we were learning back to work with us? How could we appropriately apply to our working roles what we were learning about emotional experience and development? I think that these kinds of questions are particular to the experience of being a work discussion student.

Most of us in the seminar group were not working as therapists or counsellors: we were teachers, teaching assistants, learning mentors, social workers, community link workers, nurses, and mental health workers. We were not necessarily considering changing our jobs or embarking on a clinical training; rather, we were trying to think about our work in a psychoanalytically informed way in order to enhance our understanding as well as our enjoyment of our work. However, in the excitement of exploring the emotional dimension of familiar working worlds, it was sometimes easy to devalue one's own professional role and take on an idea of a somewhat idealized therapist position, trying out some of the thinking and ideas picked up in the seminar in an undigested way that jarred with the actual remit of our jobs. While we were waking up to the unconscious reverberations at organizational and personal levels of ordinary events, such as the end of term or an absent teacher, talking zealously to colleagues about this could be counterproductive. Relationships with individuals or groups of children could also get stirred up in unhelpful ways if we failed to hold on to a realistic view of the limits of context and role. It could be difficult to stick with the value of each of our working roles and to find a way within this of making use of emotional understanding.

Learning to think about rather than to verbalize what we might be noticing was one way of managing this problem of appropriateness. In the seminar, we grew increasingly keen to translate what was described into the language of unconscious meaning. Few of us were in posts where it would have been useful to put this into words at work, but keeping possible unconscious meanings in mind could help to inform the way in which we took up the roles that we did have. As a teaching assistant, reflecting on the upheaval in a classroom precipitated by the arrival of a supply teacher, keeping in mind the children's possible unrecognized fears and worries about what had happened to their permanent teacher and what they had done to her to make her go away, as well as the range of difficult feelings connected to being a replacement teacher, could help with being more able to support both the children and the supply teacher rather than slipping into taking sides.

It could be particularly difficult to keep our thoughts to ourselves at work when becoming aware that the way in which children were relating to us or to our role might be informed by internally driven ways of relating; that how we were seen by the children we worked with might have something to do with their internal, emotional situations as much as with the external situation. Thinking in the transference rather than speaking it also provided a helpful brake on what could otherwise become a reductive, mechanical approach to understanding the meaning of what was being shown or communicated. In the seminar we sometimes became quite slick in finding transference meanings—something that could then easily become an end in itself. The temptation to sew things up neatly, quickly, and at an intellectual distance could be great; sticking with the intimate discomfort of not understanding what was observed or its impact on us could be a considerably less seductive option.

Considering the institutional context within which we exercised our individual working roles was a key part of trying to understand our own positions within organizations and the link between organizational and interpersonal dynamics. I think a critical function of the work discussion seminar is to highlight and explore this link between the individual, the group, and the institution, which promotes an understanding of and sense of responsibility for one's working role.

"Something we can use"

There are other opportunities for taking a psychoanalytically informed look at working roles and relationships, such as within personal analysis, individual or group therapy, group relations events, and clinical supervision for those doing clinical work. However, the job of a work discussion seminar is not to focus on the dynamics within the seminar group, nor to investigate the unconscious processes at work within individual seminar members, nor to treat seminars as clinical supervision groups.

I came to learn more about the usefulness of a work discussion approach when I was in the position of starting a discussion group for the nursery staff in a primary school. I was working in this school as a child psychotherapist, and it had become clear that there was a great deal of concern about what were felt to be the overwhelming emotional needs of the younger children in the school and their families. I had spent time observing in the nursery prior to the first group meeting and had been impressed with the sensitivity of the staff and struck by the high level of disturbance and need among the children. The group was not set up as a work discussion group as such, though it was a group set up to discuss work with children and parents in the nursery facilitated by an assistant therapist and myself.

In the first group, members raised their hopes for the meetings, which included wanting to have open discussions, to have a fresh look at the children's emotional needs, to join up the thinking in the staff group, to think about difficulties in engaging parents, and to counteract a feeling of being deskilled and isolated. The group suggested that if the meetings were working in the way that they wanted, then they would be more able to focus on the needs of individual children both inside and outside the meetings, there would be a sense of difficulties being out in the open and shared, and the staff would be working together and feeling less isolated and would be less burdened by stress.

In the next couple of meetings, the group tried to talk about their worries about individual children: these were children where child protection issues loomed large. However, discussion seemed to be inhibited and fragmented, with a great deal of uncertainty about what it was appropriate to talk about in this kind of group. My co-facilitator, Ruth, and I were left with a powerful sense of urgency, while remaining largely in the dark about what the staff's worries were. Doubts were raised about the value of thinking about any individual child when this was a nursery with 80 children on its register.

> One of the nursery teachers, Naomi, talked about it being hard to concentrate on just one child, or a couple of children: that there

seemed to be so much, so many—she gestured widely—and that they did need to think about the children and find strategies, and it seemed like talking about just one wasn't really going to get anywhere. I wondered whether Naomi was pointing to something that others had also raised previously, which was the awareness of the 80 children in their care, many of whom had difficulties, and how difficult it was to decide to concentrate on one child even for a short time without feeling that 79 children were being neglected. Josie, a nursery nurse, suggested that we could think about all the children one by one. Ruth and I talked about the real wish to think about all the children in turn, which we could do if we had 80 weeks—there were smiles and a slight decrease in tension—and the question about whether focusing on a few children could help. Claudia said that when they had tried to talk about a child in previous meetings, they had not really given Ruth or me any information. There was nodding, and we all commented on how in both our meetings so far Ruth and I were not included in the information loop and that also in the nursery there were different information loops, personal and professional, that people felt in or out of. There were some smiles and an awkward silence; Mary nodded emphatically. I said something about the discomfort for the group of noticing this. Most of the group then talked about the complexity and pressures of nursery life and the different roles that people have to juggle. Ruth wondered whether there was a wish for her and me to be actually in the nursery with them, so that we could experience exactly what they did. This was met with a flurry of indignation and frustration about Ruth and me not really knowing what it's like in the nursery. Claudia suggested that we should come into the nursery more often, and Mary said angrily that we should be there, otherwise we can't know what it's like. There was a gathering of murmurings that became quite heated. I referred to what Ruth had wondered and added to this that it seemed hard to feel that we in this meeting could understand anything at all about the children or what it's like working in the nursery unless we were all in exactly the same position together. Mary said, "Yes!" There was a brief pause.

There was a strong sense of hopelessness: an idea that nothing could help that was not another pair of hands on deck. After a while it emerged that there was tremendous anxiety about how the staff were working as a team and about how individual team members might be at the receiving end of blame or criticism.

> Trying to talk about team dynamics directly seemed only to exacerbate feelings of persecution. We continued to consider the problem of how to use the group meetings, the scope and limitations of such a group, the worries about what could be talked about in a helpful rather than blaming way and the concerns about protecting confidentiality in terms of both the children and the staff group. It seemed that ordinary anxieties and rivalries stirred up by feeling under scrutiny were exacerbated when all group members not only came from the same workplace but also had similar or overlapping roles within this.

Although a discussion group had been strongly wished for, it was now felt to be a rather unhelpful additional burden, increasing the pressure on staff time and forcing them to feel guilty about the difficulty in getting discussion going. Ruth and I thought that the meetings needed something outside the facilitator/staff positions, something to look at and think about that had a separate existence, though something that we could all relate to, in order to open up discussion. With some trepidation, anxious that we were creating more work for the group and unsure about what Ruth and I might be taking on, as running a work discussion group was new for both of us, we introduced the idea of modelling the meetings along work discussion lines, using observational descriptions as a way of starting to think about the emotional meaning of the observed behaviour and interactions. The initial response was a forceful protest about being expected to do yet more writing. Ruth and I asked about the writing that was already expected: it turned out that all members of the nursery staff regularly made brief records of their observations of children's behaviour and interactions. Suddenly there was an idea that rather than imposing something extra and onerous on over-stretched staff with these discussion meetings, we were talking about making use of their skills in an ordinary way; that what they routinely did as part of their work in the nursery could be valuable in developing a different kind of thinking. The group members, including Ruth and me, now seemed tentatively hopeful.

The question of whether this kind of discussion group is helpful or depriving was sharply debated in the early life of the nursery staff group and has resurfaced when work pressures are intense. In part this dilemma seems integral to a work discussion group that not only has a same-setting/similar-profession membership, but that also takes place at work and during work time. On the one hand, the group members value and appreciate the institution's investment in their professional development and recognition of the legitimate need for support that this represents. On the other hand, the physical and chronological proximity of the work discussion hour to the rest of the working day lends itself to feeling guilty about taking time away from children and parents in the nursery and, then, to seeing the group as the cause of deprivation. The fact that the nursery serves a population that has been chronically under-resourced exacerbates this situation. Early on in the group, after much concentrated discussion about whether a fortnightly work discussion hour could be justified, the nursery staff decided that rather than meet in one of the nursery rooms, as we started off doing, we should meet in a separate, more adult-oriented space in the main school, and they found a comfortable, appropriate room for this. They also requested a ten-minute gap after the work discussion group before starting work, in order to give themselves time to shift gear. And they established a system for ensuring that parents had plenty of reminders about the change in nursery opening time and a thoughtful explanation of and opportunity for discussion about the reason for this. These seemed important steps in protecting the helpful, learning function of the group while keeping the needs of the nursery parents and children firmly in mind.

Stepping into the role of work discussion group facilitator, I was aware of drawing a great deal on the way that I had been taught and on what I had enjoyed and found challenging as a student. I have found myself gripped by the tension between paying attention to the dynamics in the group while not setting myself up as the group's therapist; trying to help the group to stay on task while not being overly prescriptive about what can be talked about; hoping to develop a psychodynamic perspective while encouraging contributions from all points of view; aiming to foster an interest in emotional development based on trying to understand one's own emotional responses and including myself in this way of learning; and taking on board the significance of different experiences, situations, and roles while not disregarding similarities and continuities. For me, one way of trying to make sense of what happens, including my role in this, and so to manage the anxieties and conflicts that are integral to being in and facilitating a work discussion group, is to discuss it with my co-facilitator or to write down what has happened in a work discussion kind of way.

The nursery staff work discussion group has continued to meet regularly, and its existence is supported by senior school staff. The group decides which child to think about or whether to use the time to consider the impact of an OFSTED inspection, the arrival of a new intake, or a coming school holiday. In review meetings, and when I invited the group to comment on their experience of work discussion for this chapter, the nursery staff talked about finding that "the thinking about one child at a time is calming down, [the focus] helps with the overwhelmingness of things"; that "instead of glazing over on our own when we write our observations in the nursery, we get a chance to untangle the observations together"; that "we get a sense of what others have perceived, the similarities and differences". However, they have also made it clear that this focus, which includes the attention paid to their own emotional responses to the children in the nursery, can be uncomfortable and sometimes disturbing and can be experienced as coldly unsupportive if it veers off into ideas about right and wrong ways of doing things. Initially the group members expressed frustration that the discussions were not coming up with many tangible strategies or prescriptive advice to help them work with the children we were thinking about. More recently, they have said that "Even though we don't talk strategies, we come away with something we can use."

A work discussion group or seminar offers for exploration a range of different working experiences, roles, and contexts. Significant differences can also emerge within a same-setting or same-discipline group, as the nursery staff group found. There is an opportunity to get to know and appreciate the way that others experience their professional roles and settings, as well as to learn to see and develop one's own perspective. In this way, when it is functioning well, a work discussion group promotes a reflective, respectful approach to multidisciplinary, multi-agency work with children, young people, and families.

CHAPTER FOUR

Work discussion groups at work: applying the method

Emil Jackson

As we know, not all children or adolescents are able to ask for psychological help—at least not directly. We are familiar with the worrying ways in which young people can be propelled into action by their difficulties, while finding the prospect of any reflection pretty terrifying. For example, adolescents are often unaware of how much help they need; even when they are, many can't make the leap of faith necessary to get themselves to an unfamiliar outpatient setting—however young-person-friendly it might be. So, if we are serious about helping and engaging with young people, we need to build therapeutic bridges into their communities and particularly schools, where a more familiar setting might reduce anxieties sufficiently to enable them to make contact.

However, within schools, this relies on the assumption that staff are able, interested, or encouraged to develop supportive relationships with pupils whose education or emotional development is at risk. In reality, this is simply not always the case. While most teachers believe that the teacher–pupil relationship lies at the heart of learning, there is a striking absence of any significant input within initial teacher training relating to personality development, the emotional factors affecting teaching and learning, or the management of teacher–pupil relationships. For example, in a needs assessment carried out by the Brent Centre for Young People in ten secondary schools, only 12 out of

145 teachers (6.9%) reported that they had "received sufficient training in adolescent development" (Salavou, Jackson, & Oddy, 2002). It is therefore no great surprise that many school counsellors and therapists find themselves approached as if they were simply providing a depository for the badly behaved—providing only temporary relief for despairing teachers.

Sometimes the situation is even more worrying: for instance, when a pupil's rather obvious difficulties go completely unnoticed within the school. To give a vivid and sobering example of this: I heard about a pupil who had to do a piece of writing with the title: "How am I feeling." The pupil wrote about how depressed he was, how unloved he felt, and how he sometimes felt he might as well be dead. When his learning mentor came across this, she was immediately concerned, and showed it to the boy's teacher. The learning mentor asked the teacher, "What do you think about this?" The teacher read it, then re-read it. Looking up at the learning mentor, with a straight face, the teacher said: "I think I would give it a level 5." While this is quite shocking, we must take care not to become too critical of schools, as while some are certainly emotionally literate organizations, this is by no means always the case. Schools are increasingly beset by a results-driven culture, endlessly reinforced by annually published league tables. Furthermore, while there is lots of talk about pupil "inclusion", it is rare for staff to feel listened to, thought about, and contained in their work with their pupils—rather than the subject. This is a serious problem and one that urgently needs to be addressed.

Reviewing the context, structure, and setting: work discussion groups in schools

In this chapter, I describe the application and development of the work discussion method to teaching staff[1] within educational settings. In order to do this, I draw on my experience of running work discussion groups in schools and colleges. This has involved groups comprising a mix of staff within a school (learning support assistants, teachers, middle managers, school receptionists, etc.), groups for specific staff (e.g. learning support assistants), and one mixed primary/secondary school group. I will also be drawing on experience gained through running groups for middle and senior managers designed to develop leadership capacity.

Although most of us are naturally more interested in the *process* of work discussion groups—how they work, what preoccupations teachers bring, how insight gradually develops—my starting point for thinking about how work discussion groups might be established is to consider the *setting*. First, I outline some of the structural and contextual factors significant to school-based groups with teachers, as neglecting these factors is likely to jeopardize the longer-term viability of the work.

Timing and duration

One of the rather concrete—though critical—factors to consider is the timing of the group: when it will take place, how long each meeting will last, and how long the group might continue. Unlike training courses for which individual teachers may be able to negotiate occasional study leave, work discussion groups held in school need to be arranged at a time that is viable without unduly disrupting their primary teaching responsibilities.

Sometimes, when head teachers are clear about the developmental benefits, work discussion groups can be timetabled into the working week. However, this is often difficult to arrange[2] and is usually only possible for managers who have greater flexibility in their timetable.[3] Outside this, there tend to be three points in the day that are potentially viable: before or after school, or at lunch-time. In my experience, the best time for teachers is often before school, as this is the only time that they have—probably—not yet been pounced on by pupils, parents, or managers with multiple demands on their time. This before-school time can usually be extended if registration cover can be arranged for those attending. An after-school group has the advantage of offering an opportunity for teachers to process experiences that are fresh from the day, often enabling them to leave work with a somewhat clearer head. However, teachers do not always find this easy, as they are frequently caught up in work arising out of the day (e.g. meetings with pupils, parents, detentions, etc.). Groups run at lunch-time are usually limited to a half-hour.

Work discussion groups can vary in length from brief groups of 30 or 45 minutes to longer groups of up to two hours. My own preference is to run groups for an hour on a weekly or fortnightly basis, as briefer or less frequent groups can impede the development of trust and cohesion within the group. Nonetheless, work discussion groups can still be very effective when offered over a lunch break or on a less frequent basis, provided they are carefully organized. When working with senior managers or head teachers, a weekly meeting time is often unrealistic, and staff have preferred to meet for longer on a less frequent basis (for example, 1.5 to 2 hours on a monthly basis).

Location

In principle, there is no reason why work discussion groups cannot take place in any room within a school. However, where particular attributes are felt to be located with certain departments or individuals, geographic location may hold broader significance. For example, in one secondary school, the groups were held within the "Inclusion" department, in a self-contained building separate from the main building of the school and housing most of the support staff. While subject teachers did attend periodically, it was noticeable that over a five-year period the group consisted predominantly of inclusion staff. Subject teachers tended instead to use it as a "crisis management group", dropping in when concerns were running high; then, as soon as they felt helped, they would just as quickly drop out. From discussions about this with staff, my impression was that the location might have inadvertently given the message that the group was *really* directed at helping "special needs" children via their support staff. Might this have been different if, for example, the groups were held somewhere like the "conference room", as was the case in other schools where membership happened to include a committed core of teaching staff?

Membership matters

Voluntary vs. compulsory membership, open vs. closed groups

I firmly believe that attendance at work discussion groups should, as far as possible, be voluntary and rooted in teachers' wish for developmental opportunities to extend their thinking and professional practice. From a contractual perspective, this can understandably feel a leap of faith for uncertain head teachers who might prefer this valuable resource to be directed at their "problem staff". However, when presented as an instruction or something remedial, the resistance to engagement in the group discussion increases dramatically. This works against the overall atmosphere in the group and is unlikely to be helpful to the individual concerned. Furthermore, at a more strategic level, if one is to have any real chance of genuinely interesting the more sceptical or disaffected teachers, it is likely to be via an organic process of peer recommendation rather than a management directive.

While voluntary attendance is preferable, this can be more problematic when teachers are specifically released from other responsibilities in order to attend. For instance, one head teacher and I had several discussions about the pros and cons of directed attendance for heads of year who were timetabled to attend on a fortnightly basis; this was particularly problematic as one head of year was openly ambivalent about the idea. One helpful approach can be to have an initial pilot period, for a term or so, which can be reviewed so that the sense of ownership, agency, and involvement is greater in anything that is subsequently agreed.

Although group membership needs sufficient stability, my own experience is that, with careful negotiation, other teachers can be enabled to "drop in" to the group to discuss a pupil or situation concerning them. Providing these "drop ins" do not become too frequent, my view is that the group can and should support the tentative interest of other staff who are not yet ready or able to commit to more frequent attendance.

Representation of management structures

Linked to this, the question of *who* attends also deserves consideration. For example, it can be difficult for teachers to risk sharing "problems" in front of managers who, they fear, might judge them harshly or use information against them. Equally, it can be anxiety-provoking for managers to expose concerns to their team for fear of it adversely affecting the perception of their competence. This was certainly the case in one school where middle managers attended for only short bursts of time, in contrast to other staff, until a group was set up specifically for heads of year, at which point their commitment increased dramatically and continues six years later. On the whole, I would suggest that good working relations between group members are much easier to establish when management hierarchies are not represented within the group membership.

Group size

To function most effectively, work discussion groups in schools ideally accommodate between four and ten members. If too many attend, it becomes difficult for everyone to participate and have a voice. There is then a greater risk that some members will fall silent and eventually withdraw. While smaller groups allow for more individualized attention, they can also increase the pressure on teachers both to attend and to bring issues for discussion. Over time, this can result in teachers feeling that they are serving the needs of the group rather than vice-versa.

Setting up the work discussion groups

The negotiation of expectations and ground rules

Given that work discussion groups in schools are almost always a new venture, it is necessary to allow for exploration and negotiation about what teachers might—or might not—want to get out of the group. While this is an evolving process, it can be helpful to offer an initial "one-off" meeting in which teachers have an opportunity to ask questions, voice concerns about their work, and hear some description of how these concerns might be addressed. This process might also require some clarification about what a work discussion group is and is not. For instance, though teachers might sometimes *choose* to share something about the more personal resonance of their work, a work discussion group needs to be clearly differentiated from a psychotherapy group. In addition to helping to orient teachers, this process also offers a brief experience of how the group and facilitator might operate and reduces ordinary anxieties about the unknown.

Another fantasy, often needing to be dispelled at an early stage, is the inevitable hope that the work discussion group—and facilitator—might somehow provide teachers with a menu of magical solutions to solve any problem. The facilitator[4] needs therefore to clarify their own role and task—for instance, that a central aspect of the task would be to help teachers develop a deeper understanding about the underlying meaning of behaviour and the emotional factors that impact on teaching and learning. In the past, I initially made an active point of emphasizing that I would not be offering "expert management solutions" or "behaviour management strategies" for dealing with difficult pupils (see Jackson, 2002). However, while teachers can sometimes feel a bit frustrated that solutions are not provided *immediately*, they do, on the whole, experience the work discussion group as providing them with extremely helpful ways of thinking about pupils or situations, out of which more effective strategies and interventions evolve organically. In view of this, I now tend to say that we could, as a group, think about how one might *manage* a situation while emphasizing that the starting point for this is thinking about what is "really" going on under the surface.

Confidentiality

Some discussion about the parameters of confidentiality is always important. Rather than simply taking the form of a mechanistic agreement not to disclose anything, it can be more helpful to explore what this might actually mean in practice. After all, one does not wish to prevent learning and thinking from being shared with others who are not able to attend the groups. At the same time, it is not helpful—and could even be harmful—for aspects of the discussion to be regurgitated without careful consideration. One way to help teachers think about this is to encourage them to ensure that nothing said outside the groups will compromise, embarrass, or be hurtful to anyone.

Teachers may also be preoccupied by the question of what might be said by the facilitator to managers or the head teacher. This is an important question that deserves open discussion with everyone involved. It is not, for example, unreasonable for a head teacher to want some sort of periodic feedback about how the groups are progressing and who is attending. It is also important not to underestimate how helpful and containing such discussions with those "sponsoring" the groups can be.

How one might respond to these issues will naturally vary. My own approach is to suggest that it is usually helpful to meet periodically with the head teacher to review the on-going development of the work but to clarify that feedback would be at a thematic level and not individually attributable. I then try to discuss with the group what feedback to offer in advance of the review meeting.

Working method

Over the past decade I have explored several different ways of running groups in schools. Initially, I tried to export the traditional method in which there is an agreed rota of presentations written up in advance of the seminar. Though this can work well, my overriding impression is that, despite the "teaching and learning" environment, teachers are resistant to putting pen to paper or to risk "being marked". I therefore tend not to ask for written material—though I encourage it when possible. Instead, I see it as an important task to help "presenters" unpack their concern in sufficient detail so that it can be thought about productively. This process of "unpacking" is a vital part of developing reflective capacities.

Another structural adjustment sometimes needed is the shift from an agreed order of presentations to a decision about what to focus on, which is taken in the group at the time. The group might therefore start with something akin to a "check in", during which everyone has the opportunity to mention any worrying pupils or other preoccupations so that a decision can be made about where to start.

Potential advantages and disadvantages of school-based work discussion groups

Teachers know each other and their pupils

One of the central differences within a school-based work discussion group is that teachers are usually familiar with each other's work and role. By extension, pupils are frequently known to others, regardless of attempts to preserve confidentiality. This difference presents a number of important advantages as well as some sensitive issues. For example, when one teacher shares particular concerns, others will be able to feed in their own experiences and knowledge, such as a pupil's family history and circumstances, the context of a class group (e.g. whether there has been a series of supply teachers), or other information relating to the student's academic ability, learning difficulties, or peer relationships.

In addition to sharing relevant *objective* circumstances or influences, group members are also able to share their *subjective* experiences of the student or class. For instance, a teacher might describe having a dreadful time with a student, feeling demoralized and isolated and believing that no one else feels the same. They might then learn, to their surprise, that others understand only too well what they have described. The discovery that one is not alone is usually a huge relief. Equally, teachers might discover that others have quite different experiences. When thought of as being part of the total picture, these differences can prove extremely illuminating and lead to a range of possible approaches. For example, a student who had suffered traumatic experiences evoked in one teacher a sense of tremendous sadness. Another was filled with rage about what the student had experienced, while a third teacher felt detached and unaffected by the student or the latter's experiences. Rather than there being one *"cor-*

rect" version of the truth, teachers could soon see how they might be getting in touch with different aspects of the student's overall experience, from loss, to rage, to the sense of something being too raw to be thought about. Thinking about different perceptions in this way can contribute to a rich and informative picture for all concerned.

Like other types of *"group"* work, teachers attending not only receive consultation and support from the facilitator but also act as supportive consultants to one another. Through this process, group members develop their thinking and understanding not only in relation to their own work, but in relation to a much wider range of issues. Over time, this can lead to a culture of peer consultation developing among teachers, thereby ensuring that the work of the work discussion group takes place increasingly in the wider context of the school. As one head teacher put it: "As the project has progressed . . . I have seen my staff growing in perception, tolerance, patience and confidence in containing and motivating challenging children. Of course, such is the collegiate nature of schools that the participants' practice in turn influences that of other staff, triggering a cascade effect, even if unconsciously" (quoted in Jackson, 2002).

Protective and preventative aspects

A work-based work discussion group has a protective and preventative function for both students and staff. In one school, for example, teachers in the group were able to identify a student who was at risk of self-harm and to ensure the latter received the help needed. Without the forum of the group, this simply might not have happened.[5] Equally, work discussion groups can protect staff members from getting drawn into potentially unhelpful or inappropriate relationships with students. For example, one teacher voiced concerns that a student was becoming overly reliant on him. With help from the group discussion, the teacher was able to think about the importance both for himself *and the student* of maintaining appropriate personal and professional boundaries.

Perhaps the most compelling benefit and outcome of work discussion is the sense of validation, being understood and accepted, that is frequently reported by group members after having shared their concerns. Indeed, a key aim of work discussion groups is *to create a forum in which workers feel able to share issues, concerns, and preoccupations that they would previously not have wanted others to know about*—for instance due to shame, fear of exposure, or possible criticism. This is especially important since it is often what we *do not* want others to know about our professional practice that leaves us feeling isolated and burdened.

Anxieties of management and group members

From the head teacher's point of view it is also important for facilitators to be aware of what a leap of faith it is for them to trust someone to work with their staff "behind closed doors". One central anxiety often generated is that the group might be used as a forum to "sound off" and complain about "bad management", seducing the facilitator into establishing some sort of subversive alternative leadership. Such concerns are understandable and important to acknowledge (and contain) from the outset.

As exciting an experience as learning can be, it can also generate anxieties as we depart from what is known and enter the realm of the unknown. It is not uncommon, therefore, for teachers to be cautious at first about what they share for fear of feeling exposed, ashamed, and open to criticism. Anxieties such as these can quite easily drive a group to be dominated by basic-assumption (Bion, 1961) and other off-task functioning and therefore deserve attention from the facilitator, especially in the early phase of the group.

Schools in crisis

The only other time when, in my experience, work discussion groups seem paradoxically impossible is when the school feels itself to be in such a state of crisis or survival mode that stopping to think cannot be countenanced. One example of this was a school in "special measures" where pupil behaviour and teacher anxiety were spiralling out of control. Despite the provision of external funding to support staff, the newly appointed head teacher was adamant that work discussion groups were to be stopped with immediate effect. Although the teachers involved were extremely upset about this, the head teacher's directive was for them to be in lessons, the playground, or policing the corridors.[6] A similar situation can arise with newly qualified teachers who are so frenetically busy and vulnerable to feeling totally overwhelmed that they dare not stop and think for fear of collapsing altogether. It is often only once the end of their first year of teaching is within sight that they dare to reflect on how close they felt to breaking down, giving up and even leaving the profession altogether.

Case examples

One of the most striking anomalies of school life is the way in which intense feelings from or towards pupils—whether positive or negative—tend to be treated as if they were taboo rather than one of the most ordinary, inevitable, and potentially creative factors at the heart of learning. This avoidance is exacerbated by the general lack of understanding about some fundamental psychoanalytic ideas concerning inter and intra-personal relationships—concepts such as projection, splitting, transference, countertransference. While largely avoiding the use of psychoanalytic terminology, an understanding of these and other concepts has gradually been introduced through case discussion. For instance, instead of ignoring our internal reactions to a pupil, I have suggested that it is often these that give us the most important information about what might be going on. Teachers have found it something of a revelation to learn about the ways in which pupils who are unable to put their thoughts or feelings into words might instead act them out and, in the process, get others to experience them for them—both to get rid of their own unwanted feelings and to communicate the way they are feeling, albeit unconsciously.

In the following section I describe some examples of how issues can be tackled and illustrate the myriad ways these groups can be used by teachers.

Managing pupil–staff attachments and separations

Issues arising from pupil–teacher relationships are frequently brought into group discussion around natural junctions in the school year, in particular around holiday breaks. The following group session, just before the Christmas break, was one such example.

> Within this work discussion group for learning support assistants (LSAs), one teacher, Sasha,[7] spoke of her concerns about a 12-year-old boy called Tony. Sasha described Tony as suffering from "extremely low self-confidence and self-esteem". He lived with his mother, who had long-standing mental health problems and had to work long hours to make ends meet, leaving her with little time or energy for her son. At school, Tony had few friends and came across as lonely and forlorn. Academically, Sasha reported that he struggled terribly and that his reading and writing were more

appropriate to the level of an 8-year-old. As a result of his learning and social difficulties he had been assigned individualized LSA support involving several hours a day with Sasha.

Sasha's description of the situation vividly conveyed her sense of pain and guilt about Tony. It was as if she felt she wasn't doing enough and that his neediness was hard to bear. Other members immediately reassured her that she was helping him enormously. Sasha was grateful for this support and spoke more specifically about how difficult it was to know *how involved* to be. "I feel so bad for him", she said passionately, "he never gets to go out and just laps up any attention I offer." There was a sense of tremendous sadness.

When I invited group members to respond, several teachers spoke about what needy children they work with and what impoverished lives they often lead. One teacher added that it can be really hard for pupils "when they realize we are teachers and not friends". Another teacher chimed in with a comment about how often they get called "Mum" by mistake. Sasha added that Tony has even asked her to take him to the movies, imitating his voice assuring her that "My Mum won't mind!"

I commented on how the discussion seemed to highlight the importance for children like Tony of having LSA input and how intensely attached pupils could become to their LSA. One teacher commented on how they had to be everything—a friend, an older sibling, a parent *and* a teacher! The atmosphere in the group seemed serious as staff reflected on their importance to their pupils.

When I asked what had prompted Sasha to share her concerns at this point, she went on to describe her work with Tony and how much his learning and social skills had been progressing. However, lately he had been awful to her, though she didn't understand why or what had changed. When asked to elaborate, Sasha said that she had recently been ill and that while she was away, Tony got into a fight and was excluded. On her return, Tony was unusually rude to her, which resulted in Sasha telling him that she felt disappointed in him for fighting and that he had let her down. Since then, he had been rejecting her efforts, refusing to work with her, and once even shouting at her to "go away" when she approached him in class. Sasha admitted she felt really hurt by this—though added that she shouldn't be affected, as she was the adult.

It was important here to acknowledge Sasha's feelings, and the ordinariness of them, as well as to open up the discussion and ask the group to reflect on why Tony's attitude might have changed. One teacher thought it was simply because he didn't like to be challenged. Another wondered whether he felt betrayed that Sasha didn't "take his side" in relation to the fight. I picked up on this sense of "betrayal" and "disappointment" and wondered about the timing of Tony's fight (while Sasha was away). The teachers got interested in this. One thought it highlighted how much support was needed and how quickly things deteriorated without it. Another picked up on how Sasha had experienced what had happened, almost as if his fight felt like a personal attack. Sasha agreed, though she couldn't understand how Tony could have felt rejected by her for being away when she had been ill!

Some disgruntled comments followed this, mostly about how pupils forget that teachers are human and also need some appreciation. "They behave as if we have no feelings." I picked up on the importance of this and acknowledged how much of themselves they put into their work. I also commented on how we can all become rejecting towards others, not because we don't like them but, rather, because they might actually mean a lot. One teacher said that this was one of the difficult things about their job: when they offer themselves as a support, their pupils miss them all the more when they are away. Another teacher chuckled as she told us how horrible she is to her husband on his return from work trips. Teachers then began to speculate about whether Tony was angry with Sasha for being away and how, unconsciously, through the fight, he might have been proving that he couldn't cope without her. I reminded group members that though Sasha knew she had been ill, Tony might simply have experienced her as having been preoccupied with something or someone else, leaving him feeling rather forgotten. "I wonder if that is how he feels at home", wondered a teacher.

All of this made sense to Sasha, who then remembered that Tony had said a strange thing to her: "He warned me that he was going to be friends with me right until the last day of school, when he will do something to make me hate him." At the time, Sasha was preoccupied with what he might do and felt this was a horrible thing to say. It now occurred to her that he might have said it because he was worried about what would happen when he left school.

This whole theme of attachments and separations was then linked to the approaching Christmas holidays and the range of feelings it stirs up—from anticipation to dread—especially for those who do not feel part of a happy family unit. We talked about how this can be a blind spot in schools, where staff expect everyone to be looking forward to the break without reminding themselves that for some pupils, particularly those from troubled backgrounds, school is the break from their life outside. One teacher thought this was sometimes the case for staff too, adding that "pupils usually think we come from perfect families".

This discussion enabled teachers to think about the need to give more attention to the management of separations and endings in school. It also enabled them to consider how they might prepare pupils for the forthcoming Christmas break and be aware of the range of responses they might encounter. One teacher said that after coming back from the summer holiday, one pupil she knew well behaved as if he had forgotten her altogether! She was now wondering whether it was *he* who had really felt forgotten. This resonated for others who shared comments about how easy it is for them to forget that pupils might actually appreciate them even though they don't always show it.

As the meeting came to an end, Sasha thanked group members for their support and said that she felt much better. She added that she now understood more about why Tony had been horrible to her and how difficult it must be for him at home if he feels his mother is preoccupied and unavailable, even though it may not be her fault.

Understanding adolescence

Given the age range of secondary-school pupils, it is not surprising that many issues raised relate to difficulties experienced during this transitional period. Sufficient space to discuss these is especially important because the very nature of adolescent concerns often evokes feelings of embarrassment or shame in those around them.

One such example took place when teachers asked for help with Charlie. Charlie had just turned 13 and was described as being disruptive and disturbing to those around him. His art teacher, a young woman who was new to the profession, started off by cautiously admitting that she dreaded having to teach him. She described how, in one lesson, Charlie had made a clay penis and then paraded it around the class, using it to prod some girls and get laughs out of the boys. When the teacher wasn't looking, he then placed it on her desk, causing the class to roar with laughter at her shock. Although the incident had happened a few weeks earlier, the teacher said she still felt upset and embarrassed about it.

Group members listened and nodded. One of the older and experienced female teachers then said that this pupil also made unpleasant sexualized comments in her lessons, some of which were of a pornographic nature. She hadn't felt able to tell anyone before. Both teachers felt isolated in their respective experiences and believed they *should* have known how to deal with it. Both also confessed to wishing that Charlie would be excluded.

When asked about his home life, neither teacher knew much. Another teacher said that Charlie was an only child and that she knew his mother had recently started a new relationship. Someone else said that there had previously been concerns about whether his mother could maintain appropriate boundaries with Charlie or whether he was over-exposed to her sexual life, particularly as they lived in a one bedroom flat. Charlie apparently had no contact with his father.

It was then possible for me to raise some questions such as: why might someone behave in this way? What might Charlie be saying through his behaviour? What might we understand from the way Charlie makes others feel? How might it feel to be Charlie? The group quickly engaged with these questions and could contemplate how unsettled Charlie might feel by his mother's new relationship and sexual life, especially at a time when so much was changing for him. Perhaps he, like his teachers, felt rather isolated and afraid of sharing his worries for fear of what others might say.

Both teachers felt relieved at having aired their concerns and of having these met with a receptive and non-judgemental response.

> Having a space to think in this way seemed to serve a number of different functions. It provided an opportunity for teachers to notice and put into words how they were feeling, something they had not felt able to do before. Making sense of his impact on them also led to thoughts about how Charlie might be feeling. This different perspective transformed some of the teachers' upset, anger and disturbance into a renewed wish to help him along with a determination not to give up or "solve it" through exclusion. While I cautioned teachers against any unprocessed regurgitation of our discussion, teachers did begin to formulate a number of possible approaches including: ignoring his behaviour (which now felt possible); calling a meeting with his mother; or having a quiet word with him, at an appropriate moment, to acknowledge what a lot seems to be going on and whether he might find it helpful to talk with someone. By the end of this meeting the art teacher admitted how much she had wanted to make a scathing remark to cut Charlie down to size. She was glad she hadn't as she thought he was probably only too vulnerable to humiliation.

A couple of years later I bumped into the art teacher who, at the end of a brief conversation, reiterated her gratitude. "Thanks again for helping me . . . you really saved my life last year when I was dealing with Charlie!"

Managing anxieties and hostilities

Many discussions highlight the intense anxieties and, at times, hostility that pupils can evoke in their teachers as well as each other.

> In one group, a teacher who had recently taken over a class spoke of the difficult time she was having with two 15-year-old girls in her tutor group, Sarah and Emma. The teacher described how nasty and cruel these girls could be, laughing about her when she was within earshot and telling her she isn't their real teacher . . . she is "just a visitor". The teacher said it was like when she was bullied at school and admitted feeling intimidated. They even made her feel paranoid about what they might do to embarrass her in class. She found it "soul-destroying", and she felt "demoralized".
>
> As the teacher described the situation, her colleague interjected energetically: "I know those girls . . . that is exactly what they

> are like. They are awful . . . a bunch of hormonal, bitchy, nasty, vicious girls." The chuckles around the room indicated he wasn't alone in his view. "I've had awful thoughts about them", another teacher agreed. "Once I saw Sarah crying, and I thought: good, I'm glad you're crying. Now you know what it's like!" Someone else added, "I'm so glad you said that. . . . I always feel bad about some of the things that I think." He then mimicked a stroppy adolescent's persona, while saying, "Emma, no wonder you are so miserable . . . your younger sister *so* got the looks in your family!" The group laughed.

It is important for the facilitator to appreciate and allow for some open expression of the ordinary anxieties, hostility, and persecution evoked by the intensive and challenging nature of the teaching role, especially when working with large classes of adolescent pupils. In this respect, it is vital to differentiate between teachers simply "venting their frustrations" or "slagging off pupils" in the staff room and the work discussion context in which teachers might, at times, let off steam *in the spirit of thinking*.

Within this group discussion, it was therefore first necessary to acknowledge and normalize the level of feeling these girls generated. Only then, after teachers felt that *they* had been taken seriously, was it possible to draw the group back to the pupils' situation.

> The discussion then opened up and questions were asked about what was going on in the class as a whole. We learnt that the girls had been in the same class for four years and that they always had an air of superiority whenever they were together. One teacher commented on how they behaved a bit like gang leaders. Another wondered, light-heartedly, whether we were behaving a bit like that too, ganging up on the adolescents! This comment enabled me to ask the group what they thought might make pupils—or any of us, for that matter—gang up in this way. Group members responded readily with comments about how this happens when people feel insecure and then seek power in numbers. They were also interested when I commented on how in gangs, or gang states of mind, there is little tolerance for differences between individuals. Teachers agreed that, especially in adolescent groups, differences are frequently felt to be dangerous and to put one at risk of exclusion.[7] At this point, the teacher who had initially raised

> the issue suddenly remembered that the girls were furious that they might be moved into different classes to separate them and give the class a break. "Then *they* might feel like *visitors*", another teacher added.
>
> Gradually, teachers grew more interested in what was driving the girls' behaviour and seemed less dominated by their fear or hostility. The atmosphere shifted significantly when I asked what people thought it might feel like to be one of them. "Awful" someone immediately said. "Miserable and depressing" added another. "It must be hard work being that nasty all the time." A third teacher thought "They are really the insecure ones.... Imagine if they got moved into other classes and didn't have each other ... they'd be terrified ... especially when they know everyone hates them."
>
> At this point, the teacher who had raised the issue said something different: "Actually, the girls are not nasty all the time. When they are on their own and not with each other, they are like different people, they can be really nice. They aren't bad kids ... it's just when they are together."

The teacher who had presented the issue now seemed to be in quite a different state of mind. She was less at the mercy of how they made her feel and with a restored sense of herself as a competent professional, more robust and confident about the prospect of facing them later in the day. The group as a whole also seemed to be in a different state of mind, more interested in the difficulties and insecurities experienced *by the girls* and less preoccupied by the way these difficulties were impacting on them. As the meeting came to an end, an important discussion got going about how, if the change of class were suggested in the right way, as a support and not simply a punishment, both girls might secretly be quite relieved, even though they would never admit it.

Re-enactments and parallel process

The task of the work discussion group is not to examine its own dynamics and process as one might within an experiential group. However, there are occasions when complex issues can become re-enacted and the atmosphere starts to feel toxic. At these times, it is important to consider whether, in order to contain anxieties and re-anchor a group to its primary task, some comment about what is happening in the "here and now" may be necessary.

> This seemed to be the case in one group in which a teacher launched angrily into complaints about something that had happened the previous week. She had been teaching a class of 14-year-olds when a fight had broken out. One boy had become threatening, lifting a chair as if to throw it at another boy, and then barged past the teacher, hurting her arm. As group members sympathized, what became clear was that the teacher's upset was not primarily about the boy or incident, but, rather, the lack of subsequent support from the school. What made her furious was that when she spoke to her manager, he seemed dismissive. "He basically told me I was over-reacting!" she said incredulously.
>
> Several group members shared her outrage. Another teacher then spoke in a different tone, saying that this boy had a difficult home life—his parents' relationship was volatile, and the pupil had witnessed his mother being beaten by his father at least once. Social Services were informed at the time but did not think there was cause for further intervention. Rather than getting interested in what their colleague was saying, another teacher retorted angrily, almost shouting: "That is all very well, but this shouldn't be allowed to happen! The boy should not be allowed to become violent, and managers need to listen to what is being said." She turned to the teacher who had raised the issue and asserted, "You should refuse to put up with it. . . . I would refuse to go back to the class until he has been seen. It isn't safe for you to be there, it's abusive!"
>
> The atmosphere in the group was, by now, tense, with several members anxious at the strength of feeling being expressed. I was also struck with how quickly the relevance of the pupil's home circumstances had been disregarded. This left the teacher who had voiced them temporarily silenced.

At a time like this, when tensions are running high, it is easy for anxieties to dominate and to drive a group off-task and into some form of basic-assumption functioning (Bion, 1961). In this session, members were drawn to take flight from the central discussion—in particular from anxiety-provoking differences between members—and to join instead in complaints against "bad management" in the school and implicitly against social services too, perhaps in an unconscious attempt to preserve the cohesion within the group. In this way, all conflict and "badness" could be located outside the group, relieving the fear that an explosion might erupt within the group.

In such moments, a carefully formulated, non-critical comment about what is happening in the "here and now" is not only containing but sometimes necessary to retrieve a group from a more "reactive" state of mind, into a more "reflective" one.

> The group seemed relieved when I acknowledged what a distressing incident this must have been and warned how, when such strong feelings are around, it would be easy for us to get into a fight, either with management or each other, rather than to think together about what is happening. It was also important to alert the group to how the experience of being over-exposed to something violent and then of feeling dismissed seemed to be repeated all over the place: with the pupil who felt his parents didn't care what it was like for him to be exposed to their violent relationship; with the teacher who felt her manager didn't care; and also with the teacher within the group who felt rather abruptly silenced after she told us about the boy's home life.

By the end of this meeting, although the teacher was still concerned about her manager's response and the need to negotiate a "reconciliation" meeting with the pupil, she had felt heard and seemed more conciliatory. Others, too, spoke about how important it is to let people know when we don't feel safe and not to carry on as if we can manage anything because we are frightened of causing a fuss.

Work discussion groups for managers

It is beyond the scope of this chapter to expand on the ways in which the work discussion method has been effectively applied to those in management positions, but over the past six years I have been increasingly involved in co-facilitating work discussion groups with head teachers and other managers. The task of these groups is to provide a forum in which managers have opportunities, together with peers, to explore issues and dilemmas facing them within their management and leadership role. Discussions are, as one might expect, wide-ranging, stimulating, and challenging in style and content. Rather than focusing primarily on pupil-related issues, they tend to address preoccupations such as line management relationships, difficulties in taking up—or being allowed to take up—authority, anxieties about delegation, relationships with other key stakeholders (e.g. governing body, local partners, etc.). Given that almost all managers report a paucity of prior training in the management of people, rather than tasks or procedures, these groups have almost invariably been welcomed as a most innovative and effective resource.

The impact of work discussion groups: evaluation

As a direct result of the work described in this chapter, work discussion groups in schools are now identified as a "model of good practice" (DfES/DoH, 2006).[8]

In feedback about the groups, teachers comment on what a relief it is to discover that they "are not alone" in struggling with a particular difficulty or dilemma. Many comment on how "good it is to get things off their chest" and how "differently they feel afterwards". Teachers report that they now "feel more confident" about their work, having felt "completely out of their depth before". For some, this has meant that "instead of hating or resenting a student, they want to try to help them again".

Overall, teachers report that work discussion groups enable them to become "much more aware" of the needs of their pupils, remain "calmer with provocative students" and "much more positive about their work". These sentiments were echoed by one head teacher who reported on the "big impact on pupil achievement as well as staff morale. . . . It has made people more tolerant, not of bad behaviour, but of the pupils themselves" (*TES*, 2002). In some cases, where workers have been faced with especially upsetting or disturbing situations—for instance, in cases where young people are suicidal or when allegations have been made against staff members—teachers have reported that the groups have "literally saved them" and "kept them sane" when they felt like "giving up" and leaving the profession. Many report that the groups have offered them some of the "most useful training they have received in their careers".

Notes

I would like to acknowledge all my colleagues at the Brent Centre for Young People and the Tavistock Clinic who have helped to develop this work. I would also like to thank the head teachers, principals, link coordinators, and staff who have attended the groups. Without their input, trust, and support, none of this work would be possible.

1. For simplicity I will be referring to all staff attending work discussion groups as teachers. This does not, in any way, intend to diminish the important differences between roles such as learning support assistant and class teacher.

2. As teachers' "non-contact" times are naturally spread across the week.

3. It is especially difficult to arrange in primary schools, since teachers tend to remain with their class groups for most, if not all, of the day.

4. Within this chapter I refer to the person leading the work discussion group in terms of a range of roles, including facilitator, psychotherapist, or consultant. Though important, an in-depth discussion of these different functions is beyond the scope of this chapter. Within a training course, this role would probably be called "seminar leader".

5. For other examples of this, see Jackson (2005).

6. Interestingly, several years later, once its future was more secure, this school contacted me to re-start discussions about what could be offered to staff.

7. For further discussion about group and gang states of mind see Canham, 2002.

8. For more quantitative evaluation of this work, see Jackson, 2008, and Warman & Jackson, 2007.

PART II

CASE STUDIES

CHAPTER FIVE

Work in educational settings

A "Struggling with manifold disillusionment": a non-directive drama therapy group for adolescents who have learning disabilities

Elizabeth Nixon

I describe the work of a drama therapy group for adolescents with learning disabilities—that is, an often non-verbal group using an often non-verbal medium. Because of all that has to be engaged with, adolescence becomes a time when disillusionment takes on a particular force. Bion (1970) describes disillusionment as being the desire to know and understand about the truth of one's own experience, on the one hand, and having an abhorrence of knowing and understanding, on the other. On many levels, the work of adolescence is disillusionment. Maturity entails tolerating the frustration of being other than what we desire.

My concern is with the difficulties faced by adolescents with a learning disability in managing the adolescent tasks. Working through these tasks is greatly complicated by the reality of being born damaged or different. To be seen to be different is bad enough, as Sinason (1992) says, but unfavourably different can feel catastrophic. The sense of being unfavourably different puts an obstacle in the way of emotional growth, to the extent that such growth depends upon relinquishing omnipotence and addressing reality. The reality of a learning-disabled adolescent is one that few would ever choose.

Valerie Sinason (1992) provides us with the notion of "secondary handicap" to help us to think about that spoiling of our basic inheritance against which we all struggle, but which is so much more pertinent and likely when the inheritance we face seems unequal or so visibly and unfavourably not like the inheritance of a majority of people. Though we are all handicapped to a degree, as Sinason points out, "the extent of the degree is of great significance". She writes:

> Opening your eyes . . . to the realisation that you will not be an Austen, Einstein, Madonna or Picasso can be painful enough to the ordinary adolescent. Opening your eyes to admitting you look, sound, walk, talk, move or think differently from the ordinary, average person . . . takes greater reserves of courage, honesty and toleration of one's envy. [Sinason, 1992, p. 20]

Sinason talks of three particular forms of secondary handicapping that can occur. The first and perhaps mildest is where individuals exacerbate the original handicap to keep the world happy with them—that is, behaving like "smiling pets" for fear of offending the people they are dependent upon. This mild secondary handicapping nonetheless involves a denial of actual capacities. She talks, secondly, of a secondary handicap where the hatred of the disability and the envy provoked by it result in severe personality maldevelopment. For example, the disturbance caused by the original handicap amalgamates around a symptom, such as a harmful behaviour towards oneself or others, which provides a home for the hatred or envy. This symptom or behaviour can so readily become the focus of what others pay attention to, steering attention away from the pain of the primary handicap. This type of secondary handicap alters the capacities of a person in a most powerfully damaging way. Then there is the secondary handicapping where not thinking, being "stupid with grief", serves as a defence against trauma. In an attempt to protect the self from unbearable loss and trauma—and learning disability always involves loss and trauma to some degree—an individual spoils the capacity for thought. The secondary handicap, not the primary handicap, can therefore severely reduce intellectual capacities.

I wish to explore how and to what extent the burden of being different in an unfavourable way could be explored and named within a drama therapy group run for adolescents with learning disabilities. The thought was that by finding ways of acknowledging the pain involved in being unfavourably different, there could be some reduction in or prevention of the spoiling of the abilities and capacities that the young people possessed. The dilemma facing us was how to begin to lift the veil on what had been so understandably and painstakingly avoided and to retain faith that any good would come of it.

I would like to suggest that drama therapy provided the group with a means to explore internal and external conflicts precisely because it used the medium, which is neither inner nor outer reality. "The paradox of drama is to be and not to be simultaneously", says Landy (1993). It is possible to lift the veil on what you have been at pains not to know, as long as you can retain this paradox.

This is the story of one group's struggle to achieve some measure of disillusionment.

The group

The group I describe was made up of eight adolescents, all of whom had a learning disability. The drama therapy sessions took place as part of a special needs course within a mainstream tertiary college. The special needs course was a full-time course and was intended primarily for young people between the ages of 16 and 20 who had moderate to severe learning disabilities. All had attended special schools throughout their primary and secondary education.

The work is different from the therapeutic work normally described in therapeutic literature where the clients have been identified as having emotional problems. This group of young people found themselves in drama therapy because of tutors who believed that the young people needed a space apart to "get things off their chests". In particular, there was recognition of the "load" the young people carried in managing the demands of the college, their families, and their identity as teenagers. There was also some awareness that this group, which moved through the college—and they did just that for the most part, moved visibly as a group—carried something for the college. This group of students carried the disability for the college.

The group members were Sheila, Alan, Dipesh, Sangita, Amit, Lily, Peter, and Daniel; their ages varied from 17 to 19 years.

1. *Sheila,* white and British, was one of the two most able in the group. She was the only one able to travel to and from college independently at the start of the course. She was considered to be somewhat of a leader in the group and was looked to to put things into words—though she didn't talk a lot and preferred doing to talking.
2. *Alan,* white and British, walked around with a puzzled expression. He was often confused about what he was feeling or thinking

and would have angry outbursts where he pushed and hit out at selected male members of the group. This often occurred in unstructured situations, such as break times, or often when they had been "out in the community" carrying out tasks.

3. *Dipesh,* black and of Indian background, rushed from place to place. He spoke in two- or three-word bursts, but his speech was not clear, and he preferred to use noises to communicate with the others. He was the humorous one in the group and worked to pull the group together.
4. *Sangita,* black and of Indian background, was considered to be an extremely vulnerable young woman who had 1:1 support in order to take her place on the course. There was concern that she would behave inappropriately and put herself in danger. Her mother had died prior to the start of the course.
5. *Amit,* black and of Indian background, dressed very smartly. When he spoke, it was in quick bursts. He was generally silent around adults but became animated and excited with his friends.
6. *Lily,* white and British, did everything very slowly and somewhat clumsily. She spoke in one- or two-word bursts, and her speech was not clear. She could see to most of her personal needs herself but needed a lot more time than any of the others. She would make two or three attempts to put her bag on her shoulder or to put her coat on.
7. *Peter,* white and British, stood out in the group in several ways. He often looked as if he were falling apart: his shoes might be undone, his trousers falling down, spilt drinks and food often marked his clothes. He bumped into things, and he rushed everywhere. He made himself part of the group by clowning for them. He could speak in two- or three-word bursts. It was difficult to understand what he said.
8. *Daniel,* white and British, looked and dressed like the students on the mainstream courses. The only clue to any difficulty that he might have was the way he walked around with his head in the air, looking confused and lost. He was the most articulate of the group and could read and write.

Discovering the nature of the task

The room was set out so that non-directive drama therapy might take place. Boxes of props and materials were available at the side of the room. I set out a circle of chairs, which in the early days of the group became a sort of battleground. In the first few months, the group rarely sat in the circle as a whole group. A few members would sit in the circle at the start of sessions, and the circle would reform mainly when there had been a sort of crisis in the drama, when the play had reached its saturation point.

Initially I felt failure at their refusal of the circle: it was as if there were an unspoken and unacknowledged battle between us on this. I felt attacked and in a bind. I felt, on the one hand, that I was stupid to even contemplate that they could want to use this circle to make sense of things as a group. On the other hand, I felt convinced that the circle could become benevolent and that to take it away was to denigrate the group members. In the early days, the only thing I really had faith in was the thought that if the group was to use drama therapeutically, I had to be able to withstand attack and be prepared to discover the nature of the task. What I was to experience, in order for the medium to be pliable and flexible enough, was an enormous amount of anxiety. There was a natural enthusiasm for giving vent to inner and outer conflicts. This was immediately obvious in the way the group members rushed to the sessions. This was then followed by a surge of anxiety in response to having pushed out unwanted feelings and thoughts. I had to go through the experience of countertransference. There was no short cut. The circle, with its implicit call to come and acknowledge ownership and responsibility, seemed to be experienced as overwhelmingly daunting. For this drama to work as therapy, I had to bear witness and survive attack. Within that first half-term I experienced the task as being to be filled with rage and not to retaliate; to be attacked and not to be killed off; to be filled with powerlessness and not to become disabled; to be filled with mess and not to lose faith in the work; and to be filled with confusion and not to stop thinking. What characterized these early sessions was a mass refusal to let me speak, a huge amount of noise, and a tendency for the play to break down, the drama to collapse.

There are no short cuts

The main theme became "excluded". I felt excluded, not useful, not up to it. In the second session, members of the group used a screen to create a house. This house reappeared for much of the first year. The house was used, I felt, to create a space of their own and to provide a means of rebelling against me in a normal adolescent way. The house had all the trappings of an innocent creation and was used both as the attack and as the "screen" against the attack and the murderous feelings they had towards me, which were communicated through the noise and facial gestures. In order for them to be able to create a symbol for "excluded", I had to bear witness, be still, and not retaliate.

> *Year 1, Session 5: two sessions before the first half-term break*
>
> When I arrived in the building, I was once again met by the sight of the group standing at the door of the room. Daniel and Sheila were jumping up at the windows, and Dipesh and Sangita were banging loudly on the door. I realized that somehow the notion of an agreed start time was unmanageable.
>
> Sangita mentioned the looming half-term break. The session began with Sangita, Peter, Lily, and Dipesh sitting in the circle and Amit sitting on the edge. Sheila, on behalf of Alan, Daniel, and herself, said, "We're dressing up straight away, there's no time to waste."
>
> They then created a house for themselves, which the others kept going to visit. Daniel then had an idea, which seemed to excite them. He took some paper and wrote a large sign: "Keep Out." What followed was an eviction scene. Dipesh mainly played the role of the police, at times trying to protect the evicted demonstrating outside the house, at times being the police telling them they had to leave.
>
> Amit wavered. At one point he was inside the house and gleefully shouting protests about leaving his house alone. The next he stood helplessly outside the house, seeming unsure about where he belonged. . . .

The quality of concentration and the intensity of the involvement are difficult to convey. What is significant is that, even for Amit, who is carrying the "unsure where he belonged", it was as if having the "unsure where he belonged" as a role, held within the drama, was satisfying in some way.

They are exploring the many aspects of exclusion, and this eviction scene is a powerful symbol for them. They feel shut out for no clear reason. It seems arbitrary who is in and who is out. There is obviously a great deal of satisfaction to be gained from finding such a suitable symbol for how they feel, and it is especially exciting when you are on the inside, excluding the others. Or is it?

What I attempt to do when the play does not hold is to use words to try to contain the experience. But on many occasions the words cannot hold the experience. I am the one who has a lot of learning to do about this experience of "exclusion" before I can use words to name it.

What I realize over the next sessions is that this "excluded" is more than feeling not invited or not important enough: it is, very literally, not wanted. It seems more accurately summed up by, "Go away, do not exist. Cease to be." I have to experience it before words can be helpful. All breaks are provocations. Like all real-life events, they mobilize feelings. The experience of being "not wanted" or "excluded" is exacerbated by the half-term break, through which it seems to become externally confirmed. The imposition of a start time seems to be evidence of how much I do not want them. The session after the half-term break impresses upon me that countertransference must really be felt.

Year 1, Session 8: after the first half-term break

I arrived at the room 10 minutes before the session and was relieved not to find them in the corridor, demanding to come in.

As I got to the door, I could not believe my senses. The lights were on, music was playing, and I opened the door on what looked like a party. I was thrown. My only response was to ask how they had got in. Daniel and Sheila took it in turns to own up, and the others were busily getting on. It seemed of no import to the group, and it was difficult to speak with the music on. As I sat down, Peter and Sangita huddled close to each other. I felt compelled to sit and take it. I was full of rage. This is when I made a decision. This was an attack on the boundaries of the therapy. If we were going to have a therapy group, I needed to respond. I acted. I got up and stopped the music. I felt that I needed to speak.

I needed to say that there was a time to start and end the sessions and that it was not possible for them to come in and start the session on their own.

I was met with fury, rage, and threats. Alan and Daniel said that they were going to walk out. Sheila said that yes, she was going to down tools. Sangita wanted to know what was going on. Dipesh and Amit were practically sitting on my lap, with Peter leaning on Dipesh. Lily said, "Me too", and it was completely

> possible that she could have been seconding every point of view expressed.
>
> It felt very possible that they would leave, and I suddenly decided that they had to be given the right to make this choice—just as I had the right and responsibility to insist on the boundaries.
>
> Daniel voiced it: "You don't want us here, we are not welcome, we won't stay where we aren't welcome."
>
> "Just give us more time", said Sheila.
>
> The only thing I was sure of was that I had to stay with this. I had *done* enough: I had acted. Now I had to hold on.
>
> "Speak, speak", said Daniel, bringing a small coffee table out and standing on it. "Don't you feel stupid?" he asked, jabbing his finger towards me. "It's a trap, don't you feel stupid? They all like me. It's just you—you don't. Say you're sorry. Everyone was happy before you came in", he continued.
>
> He got down off the table and came over and patted my head. I felt as if the complete range of emotions had been experienced, and now I was almost overwhelmed by the sadness—which seemed to have been completely hidden by the rage and anger.
>
> I managed to say that it seemed it felt like having to wait to come in had made them feel not wanted. Not being wanted was the strongest feeling. It had been made worse by the break.
>
> The mood in the room suddenly changed, and postures relaxed. Daniel got up, stood in front of me, and, almost touching my face with his jabbing finger, said, "Now don't you feel stupid?"
>
> I said that what I felt most was threatened. I only realized the enormity of the "threatened" as I spoke. He sat down, and the group looked at each other.

What the session shows most clearly is that stupidity is equated almost completely with exclusion. As it takes place, it is a playing out, an exploration of being "excluded" or "not wanted", and the hatred and rage are murderous. It is only after the exchange, the non-retaliation, the survival, when I was able to show anger without murder, to show how inner and outer are different and yet related, that we could begin as a group to bear ambivalent feelings.

I used words to make sense of the situation. First of all I used the words to say how I understood what they were feeling, and why. "I managed to say that it seemed it felt like having to wait to come in had made them feel not wanted. Not being wanted was the strongest feeling. It had been made worse by the break." But this was not sufficient for the task. Daniel persisted, and in questioning whether I *feel* stupid, he reminded me that the words that came from my head would not do. I decided to use words that sprang directly from my physical–emotional experience—the countertransference. "I said that what I felt most was threatened. I only realized the enormity of the 'threatened' as I spoke."

In doing this, I was making it possible for the connections between, stupidity, exclusion, and threat to be explored, to be seen to be happening inside me. At this point it could begin to be introjected by the group. Alvarez (1992) writes that to "be able to manage what Americans call "getting his mind round it" and find the thought thinkable", a patient might first need "to explore it and examine it from a perspective or location that makes it viewable or examinable".

It is at this point—though I was not fully aware of it at the time—that my comments were useful precisely because they had the quality of drama. My comments as fed by the countertransference feelings permitted a perspective or distance to be achieved, which made an exploration of the situation possible.

I will add here that this was the first time that I felt my speech was needed, that the group wanted this. At the same time I began to be aware of the paucity of my words. The actual words spoken seemed to refer to so little of what had occurred because, as I said them, I felt and I wished to convey so much more.

Though I am unsure as to why my words felt so inadequate, which might be because of the nature of language itself or because of the experience of language for a person with a learning disability, there was a sense of validation as well.

I got the impression on this occasion, and on many occasions after this, that it was as if what my words conveyed was *also the so much more that we had just jointly experienced non-verbally*. This remains true even though the words themselves seemed so few and so flat. In the session, the point at which I say "threatened" conveys something of what I am trying to allude to. What is present in the room for all of us is the threat, which includes the stupidity and the exclusion. We have all felt it, and now it has a name: I can say it, and they can hear it. We have all shared it. We have survived. It is bearable. The group is then able to move on.

Separation

The struggle to be separate is under way. It is exceptionally painful, but for each of them it will be a different experience. When they return from the long summer break, it seems the group wants to push forward with the issue of whether separation can be achieved or whether they are damaged irreparably and forever dependent. My sense is that we can continue with such issues precisely because symbolic communication has been established. Words begin to have a regular place within the sessions. Explanations are often called for with the question "Why?" Anyone can ask "Why?" It does not just have to be Sangita any more. The play or drama begins to hold on a regular basis, and Alan starts to name one of the functions of the group. He leaves some dressing-up trousers at the end of a session and says he is putting them into the "dry-cleaners": he collects them from the bag in the next session and is pleased to see that they are "clean". He then goes on to do his own "laundry" in the session before half-term. The function of the group, then, is to empty out unmanageable feelings and to receive them back in a more manageable form. Through repeated encounters of this nature it becomes possible to learn to perform this process for oneself. The nature of the anxiety in this new term seems to have changed and, if anything, has deepened. It becomes hardly bearable.

> *Year 2, Session 12: after the Christmas break*
>
> The door opened and Sangita stood there, looked at me, and said, "I don't want to come to drama."
>
> I looked at her and said, "You don't want to come today; no, it feels too difficult."
>
> She smiled and said, "Yes difficult", and went to take her coat off.
>
> She came to the side of me and threw her arms round my shoulders and then pressed her face into the side of mine. She pressed with all her weight and then emitted a wail.
>
> Sheila said, "Are you crying?" and then anxiously asked, "Liz, what's she doing?"

"I think she's pressing into me"; after which Sangita pulled herself round and, grabbing my arm, lay back so that I was caught holding her.

"Now what's she doing?" asked Sheila.

"I think Sangita's seeing if I'm strong enough to hold her."

"Oh", said Sheila, relieved, as if that was the most natural answer in the world.

Sangita lifted herself up and said, "I love you."

"You have missed me and the group, Sangita, and it's been very difficult."

"Yes."

She walked away and went towards Sheila.

Peter had gone to sit next to Alan and Dipesh, but they looked very antagonistic towards him and were grunting and wailing at him.

Daniel was at the far end of the room, taking off his jumper and putting on a shirt he'd brought. He'd got tapes out of his bag. He walked across the room to take his tapes to the machine.

Sangita was putting on the blue dress, which she links with her Mum. Sheila had taken the white baby doll, wrapped it in clothes, and sat with it, hugging it to her. She was watching Dipesh, Alan, and Peter, who were using the chairs as "cars". It wasn't the usual road rage. It was more of a territory battle.

Sangita came and sat next to me with her baby doll. When I looked back, Peter had parked his "car" next to Dipesh and Alan. Amit took his "car" and parked next to Dipesh.

All four sat in a row.

Sheila came and placed her doll at my feet and went and sat back, looking across at the line-up.

Dipesh turned to Peter and said, "In Jail."

Daniel jumped up and took Peter's arms and put him in jail at the other side of the room.

Sheila jumped up and, I felt, crossed to the other side of the room to be away from the "jail".

Dipesh went back to join Amit and Sheila. Alan stood as if a body guard.

Peter shouted, "Shit!"

There was a chorus of oooh's.

Peter laughed, and Dipesh said, "In the bin."

Daniel went to the door and brought back the big plastic bin.

I wondered whether I had the stomach for this.

Peter laughed and went and sat himself in the bin.

Sheila looked disgusted and worried.

Sangita said, "What's he doing?"

"Peter's the part of the group that feels like rubbish, feels like shit", I offered.

Daniel looked at me and said, "I didn't do it."

Alan went to pull Peter out of the bin, but Peter shoved his bottom further in, laughing, and Alan pulled at Peter's shoe and it came off. Alan smelled it again and again and put it on the table.

He went to get the other one.

Sheila went and told Peter to get out of the bin.

He struggled out and said, "Thank you, Mummy", and she brought him his shoes.

Sheila and Alan were eyeballing each other and standing mid-centre as if they could have been acting or not. Then Sheila turned round and picked up a felt-tip pen and pointed it, like a gun, at Alan.

He put up his hands, and she shot him. He fell down, and Dipesh rushed across and magicked him better.

Then Sheila rushed across and picked up the parachute and began to chase Dipesh, Alan, Amit, and Peter; she made scary noises, as if a ghost.

There was lots of laughing, and then she sat down and created a tent. All except Sangita rushed in and joined her.

As they sat in a circle covered by the parachute, Sangita began to bite the baby, and as I talked about how she might be feeling, the others fell out of the parachute and were lying on the floor. They moved so that their arms were linked across each other's shoulders. It looked like a formation sky dive.

This was a session that was almost unbearable. I was aware that we were beginning to deal with the inevitable real-life separation from me. Sangita has already got that in mind and has ambivalent feelings towards me, which are very difficult for her to deal with—she believes impossible to deal with—as she enters the session. There is a sense in which it has become inevitable that growing up means dealing with separation from one's parents. It is also as if there is no going back now.

The big plastic bin sums up the essence of the anxiety, the nature of the fantasy, and the horror of the experience. It was sickening and horrific, it was cruel and sadistic, and it was pitiful and heart-breaking. It was all of this, and the different group members carried different parts of the experience; but; more than this, they began to carry it all. The drama held the experience, and in some ways it did more than that. It provided a means of owning it or owning as much as could be borne. As the group sat huddled under the parachute, the sense of shame, shock, and fear was conveyed by the silence. Sangita sat on the outside, biting away at the baby: testing out for the others in many ways, whether I can bear this level of sadism and debasement, and reminding me of the crime they were hiding from. As I make the link in words between what had occurred and the loss, pain, and isolation, they crawled out and did a formation sky dive. The potency and yet extreme vulnerability conveyed by this image was as poignant as the plastic bin had been earlier.

What I was also fascinated by within this session was the quality of Alan's sniffing of Peter's shoes. It had a reverence and yet a debasement too. I was reminded at the time of Lennie in Steinbeck's *Of Mice and Men*. It conveyed a brute strength and a fierce love; an exploitation and fierce protectiveness; an immense loneliness and isolation; courage and cowardice.

I often wondered how Peter could bear the scapegoat role he served as. That he could is partly to do with this complex relationship, which was developing in terms of how the group felt about their scapegoat. It reflected the extent to which they were acknowledging their disabilities as their own.

Separation—the baby in tow

There was more to be asked about whether separation is ever truly possible when you have a disability, and it was Peter who helped the group to express their agony.

Year 2, Session 24: two sessions before the final half-term break

Daniel had picked up the soft ball and wanted Dipesh to play football.

His coordination, like Sangita's, seemed surprisingly jerky. He found it difficult to stop the ball or direct it at Alan. I was shocked by his level of disability and was moved that he had risked showing this.

Peter had taken one of the baby dolls and was tying a ribbon around its ankle.

Sheila had got herself a "car" and was busily getting Dipesh to follow her.

Peter started to rush around the room, dragging the baby behind, and Sangita sat by me.

"What's he doing?" Sangita asked.

"I don't know", I offered, "but isn't that baby still attached?"

He pulled it close to him.

"Yes", I added, "the baby is on a cord still attached, he can pull it closer when he wants."

Sheila seemed half-excited, half-worried.

She chased after Peter to grab the doll. She untied it and gave it to Sangita. Then she tied herself to the ribbon and had Peter drag her round. Daniel became quite childlike at this point and shouted, "Me too, me too."

Sheila untied herself and gave him a go. Instead of tying the ribbon round his waist, as Sheila had done, he tied it around his head. He and Peter rushed around the room. Alan wanted a go and went to get the ribbon off Daniel. Daniel stood laughing and then saw the doll in Sangita's arms.

He rushed across and ripped it out of her arms, to which she shrieked, "Give me my baby!"

Daniel stood in the room, with the doll held aloft. He looked as though he wanted to hit out—to punish.

Sangita was pleading. He turned to Alan and said "football" and went as if to use the baby as a ball.

Sheila screamed, "NO!"

She was furious with him. She took hold of the baby doll and gave it back to Sangita.

Peter came and took it from Sangita, and she said, "What's he doing?"

I said, "This baby is very important today, he hasn't finished what he was showing us."

Peter retied the doll by the ankle and dragged it around again.

"In the bin", said Daniel.

Peter looked at Daniel, laughed, and threw the doll in the bin.

Sangita said, "What's he doing?"

"It's a rubbish baby, and it's still attached", I said.

Daniel said, "Give it me."

He took the ribbon from Peter and tugged and tugged at the doll deep in the bin.

Sheila was looking horrified. Everyone was quiet. He gave a final tug, and out came the doll's leg.

Sangita screamed.

Sheila rushed to the bin and pulled out the rest of the doll.

"It's broken", cried Sangita.

"Yes, it's a damaged baby", I said.

"Fix it, Liz, fix it, fix it please." She handed me the doll, and I held it.

It was as if a spell had been broken.

Peter, the most disabled of the group members, offers to the whole group something that makes sense of the experience of separation when you are a young person with a learning disability—you have a damaged baby self that you keep in tow.

The downside of this is that you can feel like rubbish. The plus side is that once you can recognize it, you can pull it as close or push it as far away as you want to. It also isn't completely you. Daniel tries this out, but it is untenable, and he goes on to show us that in his mind the baby is truly damaged and is rubbish and, as yet, all he can do in the face of this, is to express rage.

The session ended with a finale from Sangita and Alan:

Alan came over and sat by Sangita.

He said, "I'm sick of being a baby; I'm a man."

"I don't want to leave", said Sangita.

"I get angry", said Alan, "Life's so hard."

"I agree with Alan", said Sangita. "Life is difficult—it's hard—I don't know sometimes."

The spell seems to have broken, and it feels as if the truth is so hard to bear. There is a robustness to Alan and Sangita, which allows them to speak of their plight. Alan talks about his anger, an anger that has left him so confused in previous sessions, and he connects it to his essential plight: he is sick of being a baby, he wants to be a man.

Final thoughts

This has been the story of one group's attempt to think about what it means to be learning disabled, to name what it is to be unfavourably different. I believe that the group was able to recover areas of experience, parts of themselves that had been beyond words and, to that extent, unknown, because of two types of holding. There is the holding of the therapist. This equates to the holding of the mother who survives attack and hands back, in a more manageable form, strong and unbearable feelings. There is the holding of the drama—the symbolism. This is the holding that arises out of finding a substitute for an original situation of anxiety. It is finding a substitute that is in reality different from the original but emotionally is felt to be the same. It is discovering a means of exploring as yet unassimilable aspects of one's experience from a perspective that makes them viewable.

The working through of the many conflicts was always under pressure because of the overwhelming surges of anxiety that accompanied them. At such points, the drama broke down initially.

The ability to continue to work through the conflicts was fostered, in part, by experiencing these very breaks. A rule I insisted upon was that attacks had to be expressed in the drama. What gradually became apparent to the group members was that fantasy and reality are related but are separate. As it became clear that there was no punishment for attacks, no matter how sadistic, provided they were made within the drama, provided they were not real attacks, so the distinction between fantasy and reality grew.

It was interesting to see how Peter, initially one of the most visibly disabled members of the group, grew in importance for the group, and how his self-image changed. In the final term, he presented himself as the man reading the newspaper within the drama, and his physical appearance during the latter part of the second year changed. He looked smart. He travelled independently throughout the last term.

To work through adolescent conflicts and to begin to process the enormity of the reality of having a learning disability requires an ability to tolerate large amounts of anxiety and a capacity to hold deeply ambivalent feelings. It requires an attitude or state of mind where love and destruction can be held in mind simultaneously. The holding offered by the therapist and by the drama fostered this attitude or state of mind within this group. The drama, which was a readily accessible medium for the group, provided a means of achieving that necessary distance and perspective for exploring barely assimilable material. It was a means of arriving at that emotional experience of finding a way to express how things are, which can make it possible to bear how things are.

Nevertheless, there is no denying that "Life's so hard."

B Becoming a learning mentor in an infant school

Susannah Pabot

When I started work, this was my first experience as a learning mentor, and, at the same time, the role of learning mentor was also new to the school. Gradually, I was able to develop my role from a beginning full of uncertainty to a point at which I felt that I could contribute in a meaningful way to the school as a whole and to the well-being of some of its most vulnerable pupils and parents in particular. Here I discuss my work with one troubled young boy in detail, because his situation within the school and the ways in which I was gradually able to help him illustrate the specific problems I faced in establishing my new role.

With the support of my work discussion seminar group, I also became aware of some of the group processes and defensive patterns within the culture of the school; observing myself at work helped me to understand how my new role operated within this culture. I learned through regular supervision to understand the impact of breaks and the importance of a mindful space as a container for infantile emotions, and how to apply this to my role as learning mentor.

The small infant school—of fewer than 140 pupils—was situated in one of the most deprived areas of London, squeezed between railway tracks and two large motorways and surrounded by run-down council-housing estates. The Ofsted inspection prior to my starting in the post described its population as highly mobile. The school suffered from a frequent turnover in teaching staff, and the attainment of pupils was well below average overall. Severe behavioural issues were noted in all classrooms. On this basis, the school was included in the government's "Excellence in Clusters" scheme and was allocated a learning mentor post.

The head teacher, Mrs L, was making great efforts to turn the school around. When I arrived, my first impression was of walking into a special, hidden world: the corridors and classrooms stood in stark contrast to the school's desolate surroundings, with bright decorations on the walls and potted plants in all corners. I imagined what a strong impact this must make each day on the children and their families. Mrs L had appointed a number of young teachers and introduced a "nurture group" to address the behavioural problems. Based on "nurture group theory" (Bennathan & Boxall, 1996) as well as, loosely, on attachment theory (Bowlby), the aim of a nurture group is to give children who cannot manage in a classroom setting a separate space within the school where they are offered learning experiences in a nurturing environment. Mrs L ran this group herself for a term, albeit sporadically as her time allowed; now she decided that this was to be the learning mentor's role.

I soon grasped that the "Sunshine Group"—as the nurture group was called—held an important place within this troubled school and its head teacher's mind. The "Sunshine Room" was tucked between the school's main office and Mrs L's office and had its own garden, with a vegetable patch, play-house, and sand box—by far the brightest outside area in the school. In order to go to the toilets, the children had to pass through a glass corridor that overlooked this garden. When I started to work in the Sunshine Room, I saw that there was almost always a small child standing at the glass, longingly looking in. Yet the teachers seemed to have very mixed emotions about the "Sunshine Group": most referred to it as the "time-out place" but at the same time seemed to believe that the children were offered something good there. Strikingly, almost everyone spoke of the "Sunshine Group" as Mrs L's "baby"—I felt I was both pitied and admired for being asked to take over the task of its care.

The Department for Education and Skills (DfES) describes the role of the learning mentor as:

- Providing a complementary service that enhances existing provision in order to support learning, participation and the encouragement of social inclusion

- Developing and maintaining effective and supportive mentoring relationships with children, young people and those engaged with them
- Working within an extended range of networks and partnerships to broker support and learning opportunities, and improve the quality of services to children and young people.

[The learning mentor Functional Map: www.standards.dfes.gov.uk/learningmentors]

The induction provided by the borough taught me that my aim was to build supportive relationships with the children chosen for receiving learning mentor support, usually through one-to-one learning mentor sessions that were focused not on learning but, rather, on understanding and removing the "emotional and behavioural barriers to learning". My role was, therefore, clearly not to be a teacher, nor a special needs assistant. Yet when I started my post, I realized I was expected by Mrs L and the staff in the school to act like a teacher. This was very confusing to me until I was able to understand that making a space for this new and different role threatened the school's working system. In particular, I was to learn that giving an individual child—especially a very needy child—thoughtful, individual attention was felt to invite overwhelming and unmanageable anxiety that would endanger the survival of the school as a whole.

I remember my introduction to Martin's mother, Ms H, as my first significant experience in my new role. On the morning of my first day at the school, Mrs L rushed to me, clearly distressed, and asked me to "take over" speaking with a parent in her office. Ms H was in tears because of her son's behaviour. I was to talk to her about the Sunshine Group. These are my notes from this meeting:

> I introduce myself, and Ms H stares at me for a moment before she starts to tell me that this had been "the worst summer yet" with Martin, that she doesn't know what to do any more, that she will have to get Social Services to "take him off her". Ms H starts to cry and tells me that her 5-year-old son, Martin, hits her and his three older siblings, spits, throws his toys, and will neither eat nor sleep. Twice during the summer he told his mother that he wanted to die, and once he then tried to run out into the road front of a car. Ms H's voice is both angry and desperate.
>
> I ask if Martin is receiving any support at the moment. Ms H says that he "has a psychiatrist", whom she describes as useless

> because she won't prescribe tablets. The family also has a social worker who won't listen to Ms H's problems. Feeling helpless and at a loss myself, I begin to describe the Sunshine Group, which seems to mean nothing to Ms H. When I ask her about Martin's interests, she says that Martin doesn't like anything, doesn't like being at school, doesn't like small groups, and has no interests. She seems more receptive when I add that I would meet with her regularly to discuss Martin's progress.

I remember feeling that something unbearable was being "dumped" on me in a way that attacked my ability to make links (Bion, 1959)—perhaps, I wondered, in the same way as the Sunshine Group felt like a place where the children, whose behaviour attacked thinking in the classroom, were being "dumped" by the school.

When I spoke to Martin's teachers, I was told that Ms H was known for her emotional outbursts, which often contained verbal attacks on members of staff. No one seemed interested in listening to her, and I was advised not to "waste time" on what she said. Martin did not have a problem, I was told. Both Martin's reception and nursery teachers described a quiet, well-behaved, and accommodating child. However, when probing further, I was told that Martin "prefers to play alone". His reception teacher added that "last term Martin started to say he doesn't like himself". Staff became worried about Martin as he seemed to wander the corridors instead of going to the toilet, and they kept an eye on him for a while.

I first met 5-year-old Martin, a small, skinny boy with large brown eyes, the same day, in his classroom:

> Martin is sitting in the far corner of the group of children, quietly watching the teacher. He seems to be paying attention, but is timid about putting his hand up to answer questions. His arms and legs are held close to his body.

I sit at Martin's table during the following session. When I praise him, he responds by smiling. After playtime I join Martin's class once more.

> Martin sees me and smiles, then turns again and again as if to check if I am still there. He seems less attentive to his teacher than before. When I sit down at his table again, Martin wants me to go through his exercise with him. When another child asks me a question, Martin fidgets, then tilts his chair so that it

> is precariously balancing on an edge. When I look at him, Martin grins and tilts his chair further. I tell him not to tilt his chair and add that that is because I don't want him to hurt himself. Martin says that he wants to hurt himself and grins at me again.

I was deeply struck by how different this boy at first seemed to the boy described by his mother. And yet, within such a short time of my offering him my interested attention, he began to display indicators of the behaviour his mother had mentioned. They seemed to be just under the surface, ready to spill out and yet unseen or given no notice by the school staff. I felt deeply concerned for him and was drawn to trying to help him.

The Sunshine Group

Martin and seven other children aged between 5 and 7 years were referred to the Sunshine Group to work with me every day for half the day. Each of these children had what could be described as "emotional or behavioural barriers to learning"; most also had learning difficulties, and all were not achieving in class. I was given their class's work and was expected to teach them at their pace.

Although the children soon seemed to enjoy coming to Sunshine Room, I felt acute concern that taking them out of their classrooms regularly and for such long periods of time was not fostering their inclusion. And, because I wasn't trained as a teacher, I knew that I could not adequately address their learning needs either. And yet, when I tried to speak of my concerns to Mrs L or to the teachers, I felt I was not heard. To Mrs L, the fact that the children wanted to come with me to the Sunshine Room showed that all was well; the teachers seemed to want me simply to bring filled-out worksheets back and not to have to worry too much about the children.

While I was interested in the theoretical ideas behind the nurture group, I felt unable to contain on my own all that these most troubled children in the school brought to me, in addition to their learning needs. Martin most clearly showed me this and therefore helped me to understand why the group was not working. This is an excerpt from my notes after a group session:

> Martin is playing seated on his chair on his own, back turned to me, hitting two cars repetitively against each other. I walk up to him and see that he looks miserable, his face stony. I ask him

> gently if he would like to look at a book with me and another child. He shakes his head and turns further away, bashing cars against each other, then rubbing them, then bashing them.

I felt helpless to address Martin's strong feelings, as the other children around me also needed my attention. And yet he did not stop showing me that he wanted and needed to convey to me what was troubling him. A few months later I noted:

> When I encourage Martin to join an activity, he shakes his head and looks down at his shoes. Then he gets up and stands by the window. I notice that he is watching me, but he looks away when I turn to him. . . .
>
> "Martin, come here", I motion to him and sit down next to the dolls' house. Martin comes over and sits down next to me without looking at me. Immediately he picks up the little boy doll and starts playing with it, putting it on the roof and then making the doll fall down through the window. He puts the doll into the toilet and then presses him into a small cupboard. "It looks like he is hiding", I say, and Martin nods, then takes the doll out again and begins to climb up and down the house, using the windows. It feels to me that he is talking to me with the dolls, and that he is trying to tell me something important. But another child cries, and I go to attend to her.

At the same time, Martin's mother was reaching out to me for support that was not part of the school's working system and that I had not yet been able to incorporate into my role as learning mentor. Mrs L expected me to communicate with the children's parents only in the way a teacher might do: each child had a "star book", which went back and forth between myself and the parent and in which the child's progress was to be noted.

While most of the parents did not use their child's "star book", Ms H started a regular dialogue with me, filling in detailed notes about Martin's life at home. But what she wrote was about her despair, her inability to know what to do with Martin: "He kicked me today. Said he hates his Mum. Won't eat. . . ." However, both Mrs L and Martin's teacher discouraged me from meeting with Mrs H; even the support staff frowned when they saw me speak with her in the corridor. It felt as if everyone was terrified to let any of this family's distress within the boundaries of the school.

My concern for Martin and his family mounted as the months passed:

> Martin seemed very upset in the Sunshine Room today. He didn't want to participate in our drawing activity. He said: "I don't want to come to school. I hate school. I don't like the Sunshine Room." He spent most of the session on his own, his head hanging. . . . Later I sat down on the sofa with Martin and asked how we could make the Sunshine Room a better place for him to come to; he said flatly: "Put up more decorations."

While I realized that my question was not helpful to him, his answer helped me to see the way in which he had come to learn his school functioned.

I began to ask myself, with the support of my work discussion group, what the function of the Sunshine Group was and why I felt so frustrated that I was failing the children and not fulfilling my role as a learning mentor. This school seemed to be trying to provide the children with a small world protected from the pain and deprivation of its surroundings—hence also the unusual emphasis on decorations that Martin had picked up on. But this defensive denial of the real context led the whole institution to be under great stress: for the children for whom the safe world was to be created carried the other, outside world inside them. The most vulnerable children, and their parents, with whom I as learning mentor was expected to work, could not keep their anxieties and pain from spilling out.

Hinshelwood (2002) wrote that organizations build defensive patterns against overwhelming anxiety, much as a person does. He suggested that this can be partly due to the "pressure to perform a visibly competent role" in the face of anxiety, and I wondered about the impact of the recent negative Ofsted report.

The school also seemed like a mother who cannot bear her infant's negative projections and is therefore unable to understand and contain his experiences—not unlike Bion's dutiful mother who responds to her infant's cries, but cannot take into her his powerful fears and emotions (Bion, 1959), for there were certainly good intentions among the staff.

The Sunshine Group was meant to provide the most vulnerable children with the most generous injection of the goodness the school could muster; but because it could not allow the bad in next to the good, all this goodness alone could be of little use or meaning to the children. The new role of the learning mentor did not fit into the school's defensive pattern of functioning, because its aim was precisely to address those aspects of the children's "barriers to learning" that the school was trying so hard to keep out.

Introducing a new kind of space

At this point I spoke—with Ms H's and also Mrs L's permission—to Martin's psychiatrist and social worker. They were eager to communicate with the school and to try to build a support network for the family. I learned that Martin's psychiatrist had been trying to convince Ms H to allow him to go to child psychotherapy sessions, but Ms H would only agree to help from the school. With the support of my work discussion tutor and in agreement with Martin's psychiatrist, I was able to speak to Mrs L about offering Martin some individual, unstructured time in the form of one-to-one learning mentor sessions, initially twice a week.

Both Martin and I approached the beginning of this new way of working with considerable anxiety, as my notes from Martin's first 1:1 session reveal:

> When I picked Martin up for his first individual session, he looked up at me immediately. I smiled and motioned for him to come with me. Martin jumped up and walked a few steps towards me, looking at me with a smile he seemed to want to hide. Then he suddenly tipped sideways—I wondered whether he had tripped, but didn't see anything on the floor in his way—he seemed to have simply lost his balance. Martin fell onto the floor and got up again quickly, looking confused. . . .
>
> Out in the corridor I said to him that we would go to the Sunshine Room using the "secret back way".

This is a route behind the main school offices that allows staff to move from one part of the school to the other without walking through the entire building, past glass-walled classrooms. I must have chosen this way that day to avoid walking past the whole school, showing everyone that I was offering Martin something different. I think my using the word "secret" arose from my considerable anxiety about the school staff's response to this new way of tackling Martin's difficulties. I knew there were objections to any child receiving individual special attention and was fearful of stirring up trouble.

Indeed, my 1:1 sessions with Martin quickly caught the attention of both children and staff. Each time I went out into the playground, a child would come up to me, begging me to take him too. Members of staff would frequently open the door while we were working, either "by accident" or even deliberately, and one teaching assistant even asked Mrs L to install a glass window in the Sunshine Room door. Martin's class teacher repeatedly gave me worksheets for him to complete in his time with me, although I explained to her that the focus of his sessions was to give him unstructured time. Often I was asked not to take him out of class during our regular times, but to come later.

During these first months Martin chose to spend much of each session simply playing board games. I felt that these games with rules and pieces to hold on to gave him a structure that made our individual time less anxiety-provoking. They also seemed to give him a sense of power, as he often tried to control the outcome of each game by taking over my turns as well as his own.

Breakdown and a new start

The six-week summer break at the end of the school year proved to be a great challenge to Martin's family. Ms H reported that Martin had been uncontrollable and had again tried to hurt himself and others in his family. He had also broken out in psoriasis over his entire body (Martin suffered from this illness, but it had never been this bad).

Martin did not come to school on the first day, nor on the second; Ms H said he refused to leave home. I suggested that Martin should come to the Sunshine Room for a session with me each day until we had worked out a support plan for him, and he then agreed to come to school. This is an excerpt from my notes after my first session with him. Martin is now 6 years old:

> When we arrived at the Sunshine Room, Martin picked up some blocks and hurled them across the carpet at the dolls' house. He was throwing them very hard. I said that Martin was showing me how angry he was. I added that it was okay for him to throw blocks, but that I would make sure he wouldn't hurt himself or me. Martin threw some more blocks, but not as hard. He was moving quickly, without making eye contact with me.
>
> Then, suddenly, Martin turned to the dolls' house and picked up two boy dolls. He made them climb up the doll house wall.

> I said that Martin had played like this before the long summer break. Martin looked into the doll house and said that a doll was missing. He started to look for it, and when he found it inside a closet, Martin smiled and said that he himself had hidden it there.

I realized how important it felt to Martin that I was able to bear his anger about the break. Bion (1962b) introduced the notion of "containment" as a troubled state of mind that is held together. When, as Waddell (1998a, p. 34) writes, "the experience has been understood, it becomes possible to express it symbolically, to learn from it and to develop beyond it." I wondered whether Martin felt that the hidden doll was an aspect of himself that he had left in the Sunshine Room, and whether finding the doll safe meant something about this part of him had been kept safe also.

I began to think about possible deeper meanings of the break for Martin. O'Shaughnessy writes that, to the baby, "the absent object is a bad object which is leaving the baby to starve and die" (1964, p. 34). Klein linked the appearance and disappearance of the good object and the mechanism of "splitting off and destroying one part of the personality under pressure of anxiety and guilt . . ." (1946, p. 20). It seemed that Martin had two very split sides within him—"good" Martin at school and "bad" Martin at home—and that this split was accentuated during the breaks, which exposed him to the absence of a good object (his school, his learning mentor).

Martin's psoriasis outbreak led me also to think about Bick's discovery (1968) that infants who do not experience early containment may develop fragile second skin functions; I wondered whether Martin's school personality functioned in this way for him, and whether the loss of school during a break led his skin, literally, to disintegrate.

I realized that there was no thinking within the school that took into account the children's feelings about breaks; when I had mentioned to teachers my own sadness about saying goodbye to the children who were leaving the school at the end of the year, they laughed at me and made comments such as: "We'll be glad to be rid of them." It struck me how difficult it was in this school, where children and staff came and went frequently, to think about gaps and absences. Martin seemed to show me how much children, particularly in schools like this one, needed to know that despite breaks they were being kept in mind.

Consolidating a redefinition of the learning mentor role

Two important decisions were made: Martin would continue to come to one-to-one sessions with me every day for half an hour and at regular times; and I would receive additional supervision from my work discussion tutor, paid for by the school's learning mentor budget.

I began to insist on protecting Martin's sessions: I made a large sign to say that while I was "in session" my door should only be opened if absolutely necessary, and I no longer accepted his session times being moved around.

Martin's teacher and the school's SENCO were able to see improvement in his learning and engagement in the classroom during the first half-term. In due course, three other children were referred for one-to-one learning mentor sessions. I continued to run the Sunshine Group, although I was now able to negotiate providing shorter sessions with younger 4- and 5-year-olds, who benefited from a small group with a focus on play rather than learning. Because I was able to offer more in-depth support to those children who needed this, I no longer felt that I was simply expected to be another teacher—I felt I was finally establishing a meaningful learning mentor role.

Another important aspect of my work was to be the person at school who "held in mind" for the child and his family all the support services outside the school. So, as the first Christmas break approached, I contacted Martin's psychiatrist and the family's social worker to find ways to support the family during this time. A place for Martin was organized in a holiday play scheme, and the social worker was able to meet Ms H during the school holiday. This is an excerpt from Martin's first New Year session with me, after this break. That morning, when Martin arrived at school with his mother, he was holding a game, and she told me that Martin had played this game with her, his siblings, and the social worker during the break:

> When I arrived at Martin's class, he seemed to have been waiting for me. He looked at me, smiled broadly, stood up, and said in a loud voice to his teacher: "I'm going to the Sunshine Room with Susannah." He sounded much more confident than I remember ever having heard him sound before, and it felt to me as if he wanted everyone to hear that he would be going to his session with me.
>
> When we arrived in the Sunshine Room, Martin paused in front of the table, holding his game. He didn't say anything, but looked

> up at me. I commented that it had been a very long time since he had come to the Sunshine Room. Martin looked down at his game. I asked him if he wanted to show me his new game. Martin nodded and smiled, and pulled out a chair to sit on. He was smiling broadly as he unpacked his game, and his legs were moving excitedly under the table. Martin said that he would be red and I yellow, and we started to play the game. We played once and then again, with Martin winning both times. It felt very important for him to win, not so much because he wanted to be in control, as I had felt previously, but because he wanted to show me what he had learned during the break.

This led me to think of O'Shaughnessy's statement (1964) that "the absent object is a spur to the development of thought".

Concluding thoughts

Martin continued to come to learning mentor sessions with me until he moved on to junior school, and, despite big changes in his family life, including the birth of a sibling, he was able to make good progress in school throughout this year.

I was able to gain confidence, largely through my work with him, that a learning mentor can make a difference to even a very troubled child within the school setting. It was clear to me that this role allowed children of parents who were not able to accept help from outside school—and in my experience many of the parents of children who were referred to learning mentor support struggled with this—to access a kind of support that had hitherto not been available within the school sphere.

There was initially considerable resistance within the school to my new role, but, as my confidence grew, I was able to see others within the school begin to think in new ways about the children, about breaks, about painful situations. It was very moving to me to see how even a small change within an institution, such as allowing a new professional role to develop, can lead to growth for the institution as a whole.

C A therapeutic approach to working with primary-school children

Suzan Sayder

> Learning depends on the capacity for [the growing container] to remain integrated and yet lose rigidity. This is the foundation of the state of mind of the individual who can retain his knowledge and experience and yet be prepared to reconstrue past experiences in a manner that enables him to be receptive of a new idea.
>
> Bion (1962a), p. 93

Background

My first work experience with children, which I undertook as part of a planned change of career, was as a volunteer in a programme called Volunteer Reading Help (VRH).

VRH is a national organization that recruits and trains volunteers from the local community to give individual help to children in primary schools. The children are selected by their teachers to participate in this programme because they are underachieving. Their difficulties are believed to be to some degree emotionally based. While the format of the sessions with the children was quite flexible, as a reading assistant I was expected to engage them in activities that promoted literacy. The children were seen individually for half-hour sessions twice weekly. The main objective was to provide them with individual adult time and attention, in the hope of boosting their sense of self-worth and, in turn, improving their academic performance.

At VRH, I felt that the organization recognized the link between cognitive learning and emotional states of mind. They make it clear in their stated goals that they aim to help children who lack confidence and are underachieving. The fundamental idea that underlies this philosophy—whether or not the founders of VRH were aware of the theoretical link—is Bion's model of "container/contained" and his corollary "theory of thinking". In essence, children may experience difficulties in learning if they are unable to internalize a self-containment function from their early experience. If the anxieties associated with learning, such as uncertainty and frustration, are too painful to think about, the child may switch off or become "mindless". As a result, the process of thinking and learning can become stalled.

Bion's concept of containment (Bion, 1962a) suggested that the mother has to be sufficiently in touch with her infant's feelings in order to make sense of them. Even if she does not immediately understand the cause of the infant's distress, she needs to be able to bear the anxiety and uncertainty.

In his theory of thinking, Bion maintained that if the infant's primitive anxieties can be digested, then his mind will develop an appetite to take in new things and, in turn, to think and to learn. Bion referred to this mode of mental functioning as K (Bion, 1967b). In essence, the capacity to think comes from being thought about. As the early mother–infant interaction sets the stage for later development, an insufficiently containing early experience may lead to difficulties in cognitive learning.

The VRH philosophy recognized the link between emotional states of mind and learning difficulties, and the potential for simulating the mother–infant containment function in a therapeutic relationship between worker and child. However, for the worker to provide containment for the child, the worker herself must feel held and contained. I now realize how isolated I was at VRH, as no formal supervision was provided by the organization. I did feel, though, that I had the full backing of the head teacher as well as on-going contact with the class teachers. I was fortunate to have the support of my work discussion group.

A therapeutic setting is meant to have what Salzberger-Wittenberg, Henry, and Osborne (1983) term "a well-defined spatial boundary" and provide "the security which derives from being held within a space and by a reliable person's watchful eyes" (p. 10). If delivered in a good-enough way, it should provide the children with a secure base for self-exploration and emotional growth.

The primary school environment seems, by its nature, to ignore the needs of the individual in some ways. For example, there are inevitable space and resource constraints. The classrooms and teachers are shared among large groups of children with competing interests and needs. Children sit and work at large tables, and their places are entirely interchangeable. Stationery supplies are often kept in the centre of each table and shared out.

I found that this communal atmosphere occasionally carried over to, and interfered with, my work with the children in my VRH role. I normally worked with the children in the school library, an attractive space with good natural light but one that was not entirely free from distraction as other children often came in and out during the sessions. On occasion, we were asked to go to a different room because the library was needed for "special" group work. These disruptions and displacements were clearly unsettling for the children. Such experiences accentuated the scarcity of individual attention and space, and the importance of the kind of individual work I was doing with the children.

By understanding the process that takes place in a good mother/infant bond, one can see how it can be mirrored in therapeutic communication. It begins with being capable of comprehending the child's anxieties as they are projected onto the worker. My task, as the worker, was to mentally digest them and offer them back in a way in which the child could understand them.

The child may project certain unbearable feelings of helplessness, confusion, disintegration, shame, or fear either from a wish to get rid of those bad feelings or in the hope of being understood and helped. If I could receive the child's communications in the right way, I could help cope with those anxieties. This in itself is the greatest challenge in this line of work. As Abrahamsen (1993) explains: "It is very painful to wait, to remain receptive, to bear the pain that is projected, including the pain of one's own uncertainty" (p. 49).

Also, I have come to appreciate the importance of boundaries in a therapeutic relationship. Copley and Forryan (1997) stress the importance of establishing a framework in terms of the setting to be able to relate to one's "client" in a reliable way and hold him or her in mind at that time and place.

At VRH, certain aspects of a therapeutic framework were encouraged by the organization—such as seeing the children at specific times and in a place designated for our work. In addition, I was careful to avoid missing sessions and tried to prepare the children for breaks (and endings) well beforehand. Also, I resisted sharing any information about myself or my family.

The children

The VRH children were selected because of their difficulties with reading. Perhaps, as suggested by Bion's "theory of thinking", there was a link between those difficulties and their early experiences. Although I did not have the opportunity to meet the families of these children or to learn about their early experiences, I wondered, as I began to get to know them, whether a good mother–infant bond had been securely established. Waddell described the container–contained interaction in infancy as "representing an emotional realization of a learning experience which becomes progressively more complex as it constantly recurs in different forms throughout mental development" (Waddell, 1998a, p. 103).

Aleke

One of the children I worked with at VRH was Aleke.[1] She was a slender, quiet girl of African descent. Her education at this school was interrupted by a two-year gap when her family moved to Gambia. I started to see her shortly after she returned to London and to this school. When I came to collect her, I often found it difficult to see her—as if she were invisible. She was virtually unable to read when I met her, aged 8, and was described by the teacher as being "rather lazy". Initially, she had three brothers, two older and one younger. Subsequently, her mother gave birth to twin boys. Each of the six children—save the twins—has a different father, none of whom lived with them.

Aleke seemed to me to be trying hard but displayed an inhibited capacity to think and learn. She shared her desire to "know things" with me when, on several occasions, she would greet me with queries about the meaning of words that had come up in class discussion. Also, she would occasionally interrupt our reading to ask me to explain the meaning of unfamiliar words. I responded by explaining what the words meant and suggested that we start a vocabulary list that we could review each week. Aleke agreed to this, but I found that, from one week to the next, she would have completely forgotten the meaning of all the words. Any mention of this list seemed to heighten her anxiety, and after several weeks I suggested that perhaps we stop keeping the list. I felt that knowledge seemed to "leak" out of Aleke, retarding her cognitive development. Copley and Forryan referred to a "sieve-like" form of non-containment, in which information cannot be taken in and hence seems to run through a person (Copley & Forryan, 1997). In retrospect, I believe I should have helped her to acknowledge her feelings about not being able to learn these words, especially after showing an interest in knowing their meaning.

Aleke's teacher reported that, although she diligently memorized her spelling words each week, she could not grasp their phonetic structure. In her spelling tests, her teacher would normally call out the words in a different order, but Aleke could only write them in the order in which she had memorized them. If the first word from the list she memorized was "train" but the teacher called out "house", she would still write "train". She was unable to comprehend the difference between the sounds. This reminded me of Bick's idea (1968) of "adhesive identification" as a rote mode of learning where no real understanding can take place, where only a two-dimensional relationship was possible because the "third dimension" was felt to be like a "fall into space", as in Bion's "nameless dread".

When we had our last session in December of the first year, Aleke left with high expectations of Christmas and the school holiday. However, when we met again in January, she talked only of the disappointments surrounding the holiday. Not only was she disappointed with her presents, but also her brothers had "fought the entire time". By contrast, she greeted me that day with unaccustomed familiarity and enthusiasm. She called me by my name, which she had not done before. She nodded and smiled broadly when I asked whether she had remembered I was coming that day. It felt very chummy, and I reflected later that I had not experienced this intimate feeling before (and did not again). I wondered whether Aleke had held on to her idea of me in perhaps an idealized way during that disappointing break. Towards the end of the session, she kept looking at the clock and remarking anxiously that our time was nearly up. I knew that she was unable to tell the time, but she seemed to have suddenly realized that our time together was not without limit. She seemed sad when we parted—a depressive kind of sadness. In her fantasy, she seemed to have held on to an unrealistic idea of our relationship; but faced with the reality of the session, she was left only with a feeling of emptiness.

Again, I wished I had done more to help her to understand her feelings. However, Aleke's projection of despair left me without words to respond to her. In working with Aleke, I was aware of powerful projections that elicited feelings of inadequacy in me. In addition to her painfully slow progress in reading, I found that Aleke smelled of body odour and believed that she must not be very well cared for. I often felt overwhelmed by my desire to teach her and to make her life better. However, in order to help Aleke at all, I needed to learn to contain her own feelings of inadequacy and her disappointment without being overwhelmed by or being in projective identification with them.

During my second year of working with Aleke, I felt that I was finally making progress. One day, during a particularly easy passage that I was reading to her, I pointed as usual to the words as I said them aloud. Suddenly, without any prompting from me, Aleke started to read too. I stopped to allow her to go on by herself, but then she stopped as well. I started again, she joined in, and we continued to read the passage together. Although she had not been able to take over the reading, I felt that I had enabled her to feel safe enough to carry on *with* me. In the months that followed, Aleke gradually began to read very simple texts on her own.

Layla

Layla, another child I worked with at VRH, was a friendly, cheerful girl whose parents came from Morocco. She was plump, had a very pretty face, and always wore a headscarf, as her family was devoutly Muslim. Layla was the youngest of six children, with one brother and four sisters. Only one sister (aged 16) still lived at home with Layla and her parents. The other siblings were married, with children of their own. Layla often mentioned members of her immediate and extended family, and they sounded very closely-knit.

When I first started to see Layla, she talked often about her family and their summer holidays in Morocco. She boasted of the many animals she had in Morocco—rabbits, dogs, cats, and horses. She also talked of happy summer memories there—playing with cousins and even having a boyfriend. It did, indeed, sound rich and wonderful. She seemed to look forward to the first summer holiday with great longing and anticipation. With all this talk about Morocco—and, conversely, little talk about England—I wondered about the experience of her parents and older siblings. Perhaps they held an idealized sense of Morocco, in contrast with less than ideal feelings about England.

Early on in my work with Layla, we read a book about a horse in the British Horse Guards Cavalry that was too spirited for the corps and was often scolded and punished. The horse is told: "Forget your feelings, it's others' lives you guard." This passage caught Layla's eye, and she said that her mother had told her to "forget her feelings" when her paternal gran had died the previous summer. I wondered if that was how her family had dealt with their own sad feelings about loss, such as the loss of their homeland. Perhaps they were unable to work through the mourning process associated with leaving Morocco because they did not allow themselves to acknowledge their own sad feelings. Freud explained that if the loss of an object—whether "one's country, liberty, an ideal" or a "loved person"—cannot be acknowledged and mourned, a melancholia or depression can ensue (Freud, 1917e[1915]). The idealization of Morocco might have provided Layla's family, and Layla, in her identification with them, with a defence against their grief.

Layla's family, being devoutly Muslim, seemed to have little tolerance for—and, in fact, seemed to disdain—Christian values associated with England. Layla became very interested, towards the end of out first year together, in a book she found in the school library called *The Muslim World*. She read the book aloud to me nearly from cover to cover, and I was struck by the way her reading seemed to be remarkably more fluid than with other books. She seemed to make a greater effort to sound out the difficult words and to ask the meaning of words she didn't understand. Initially, she had wanted to take the book home to show her family, but she said her elder brother would not allow it in the house as it showed a picture of a Christian monk. I explained that while the monk was Christian, he was included in this book because he had met Mohammed as a young man and had recognized his potential for greatness. Layla said it didn't matter, her brother would be very angry, and she did not take the book home.

I felt that Layla struggled with the conflict between her family's beliefs and her exposure to British customs. Layla seemed to hold primitive persecutory fears that the school dinners secretly contained pork because the teachers wanted to trick the Muslim children into eating the forbidden food. Several dreams she shared with me involved murderous conflicts between Christians and Muslims.

Layla once told me that she had listened in on her sister's phone calls and feared that "God would pour hot lava in [her] ear when [she] dies as a punishment for her sin." This idea of God seemed to represent a punitive superego, and I wondered whether it symbolized her parents' implicit (or explicit) warnings to her that she would be punished for opening her ears to hear "inappropriate" British or Christian things. In other words, perhaps she had an unconscious anxiety about the danger of listening to other points of view or opening her mind to different ways of thinking. As Waddell pointed out, "under the sway of anxiety, thinking becomes separated from its emotional base and irrational or rigid ideas and attitudes begin to supervene" (Waddell, 1998a, p. 12).

This led me to think about my own experience with Layla. I observed that she wanted to do all the talking. If I commented on or wondered about the things she was telling me, she did not reply. In fact, she often talked over me—as if she feared that I might brainwash her if she let my words in. I wondered about the link between this behaviour and her reading difficulties. It was as if her cognitive learning was blocked by her infantile persecutory anxieties. Once, in a moment of frustration, I pointed out to her that she did not seem to want to listen to me. I realized at the time that I had said it more forcefully than I had intended. However, my comments did seem to bring about a change, because Layla began to listen much better after that. I reflected later that perhaps she had been frustrated with the feeling that she was not being listened to at home and had projected that feeling into me.

I had the impression in working with Layla that she wanted to make better sense of the two separate worlds she lived in. I wondered if perhaps she held some hope that they could co-exist and perhaps be integrated. In our second year of working together, Layla read a story about a girl in a wheelchair. The parents of this girl were overprotective, and Layla said, "If I were her, I would tell my parents to leave me alone because I could do things for myself." Perhaps Layla saw herself as the girl in the wheelchair, handicapped by conflict but optimistic about her ability to manage on her own, if ever permitted to do so.

In the spring of our second year together, Layla told me that her father was selling their house in Morocco. She was hugely disappointed that they would not be able to have their usual holiday in Morocco that summer, and she struggled with her disappointment for many weeks. However, this event seemed to mark the beginning of a new phase for Layla. She seemed more grounded in the months that followed. Her life in England seemed to take on more importance. It was during this period that I had feedback from her class teacher that her reading had improved.

Towards the end of our time together, Layla told me that she wanted to have a birthday party and invite friends from school, but that she didn't want her brother to find out because he did not believe good Muslims should have parties. At first, her wish to keep the party a secret seemed to be an act of defiance. However, then she told me that her father had encouraged her to have the party and had said "those who want to come can come, and those who don't can stay home". Perhaps there had been a shift in the way her parents felt about their commitment to being in England, as demonstrated by their decision to sell the Moroccan house and to stay in England that summer. Her father's encouragement for her to have a party seemed to reflect a more integrated point of view.

Endings

When I knew that I would be leaving my VRH position at the end of the second school year, I felt anxious about making the ending as good as possible. I was able to announce my departure four weeks beforehand, which I hoped would give the children (and myself) enough time to reflect on what had taken place during our time together and to prepare for saying goodbye.

During those final sessions, Aleke and Kedif (the other child I saw at VRH) wanted to recall, talk about, and reread some of the same books we had read over the two years. It seemed that they needed a concrete way of trying to hold on to the experience. As Salzberger-Wittenberg pointed out,

> as external relationships come to a temporary or permanent end, [there is a] fear that one will forget as well as be forgotten and lose what has been of value. . . . Such anxiety makes students and teachers alike look for proofs of achievement and wish to embody it in something concrete. [Salzberger-Wittenberg, Henry, & Osborne, 1983, p. 153]

Only Layla, who by the end seemed the most psychologically integrated of the three children, could function more symbolically. She was able to articulate her sad feelings about our ending and tell me that she would miss me. In one of our final sessions, she commented that because so many people had left her, she thought that maybe she should lose weight. If people could see the inside, she explained, they might not leave her. I told her what I saw of the Layla inside: a clever, thoughtful, and interesting girl, whom I had enjoyed getting to know. She seemed pleased with my reply.

For the last session, I had arranged for the three children to join me on an outing to the local library. None of the children had ever been before. I wanted them to see it for themselves and to take home forms for obtaining their own library cards. The outing was pleasant and rather poignant. On the way back, Layla asked where I lived. She wanted to know my address, she said, so she would know where to find me. The others chimed in and wanted to know too. Maybe this query stemmed from fantasies about my personal life or feelings of envy about my own family. Or perhaps there was a worry that she/they would not be able to hold on to their experience with me. I did not give in to their requests, but I did agree to visit them in the new school year. I wondered about my own motives. Had I agreed to see them again to avoid confronting the real pain of separation?

I returned to the school in the autumn term for our brief pre-arranged visit. Again, I met with the three of them together. I was pleased to see how cohesive and self-sufficient they appeared to be. After a round of "news", they asked to read a book. Together, they chose a fairly simple storybook, but one that none of them had read with me before. I offered to read to them, but Layla took charge of the situation, saying they would read to me instead. She determined that the book should rotate among them, with each child reading a page at a time. At first, Aleke said she didn't want to read, but she soon gave in to Layla's insistence.

Layla's personification as a capable adult and the group's demonstration of independence initially made me feel rather useless. However, it moved me greatly to see that they were more self-reliant than before. I thought about the function of containment in a therapeutic relationship being to empower the individual to internalize the therapeutic function, allowing the relationship to move on and eventually to end. Layla asked me if I would come back to watch their Year 6 play, which would be performed in June or July. The others echoed the invitation. I said I would try to come back for that important event.

The ending of my work with these children coincided with the end of their school year and anticipation of their final year at primary school. For me, it represented the end of my work at VRH. As explained by Salmon, "the ending of one thing signals the beginning of another. The pattern is set into motion at the time of the earliest ending/beginning—birth. The way in which each ending is managed has a profound effect on the potential for further development" (Salmon, 1993). Each of the children and I myself had to "let go" of our relationship in the way we had come to know it. However, I felt that the experience had been enriching for all of us indifferent ways, and I hoped it would ease the transition to new endeavours.

For the children at VRH, I believe I provided a containment function by thinking about, and trying to understand, their anxieties. While I struggled with trying to make sense of their communications during the sessions, I think I helped them by providing a therapeutic setting and thinking about the feelings they elicited in me. As I developed my observational technique through my infant- and young child observations, I gained great insight into the value of being a receptive observer rather than "doer". In a subsequent work setting, I found I could more often name the communications in the interaction so that the child could think about and reflect upon their own experience.

D A creative arts project in a primary school: the impact of "bizarre artefacts" in the classroom

Karl Foster

"Bizarre artefacts" are the contents of a creative learning and thinking resource called an "Object Dialogue Box", made by myself and another creative practitioner. They present the learner with an unfamiliar challenge because of their unusual symbolic form. Often two everyday items are merged to form something that is not easily knowable or nameable. They become catalysts, or entry points, for other experiential learning.

I shall explore the emotional impact of the artefacts through the progress revealed in children's group narratives and in their individual written narratives and by using observational material from class sessions in a primary school.

The psychoanalytic aspect of this inquiry investigates how the desire to learn and the will to create is internalized from within the infant–mother relationship. I examine what the challenge of the artefacts represents to the internal world of the child. An adaptation of Bion's idea of "catastrophic change" (Bion, 1965, p. 8) provided the inspiration to understand what type of change the project facilitated.

> Man is always, I think, made fearful by what he does not understand. I heard the other day a story which illustrates the point and which may appeal to garden lovers. A lady wishing to keep people from crossing her lawn put up a notice BEWARE OF THE DOG. It

> had no effect. She then put one up BEWARE FIERCE DOG—still no effect—but when she put up BEWARE AGAPANTHUS no one dared come near. [Jim Ede—Founder of Kettle's Yard, Cambridge. "Open House" Exhibition Catalogue]

This quote gets at the essence of the fearful impact of the unknown.

Jim Ede recounts this vignette to help visitors to galleries to approach art and artefacts with open and creative minds, rather than expecting to find what is already known. There is a risk in embracing the unknown, the challenging, and the difficult, but without the risk there can be no development, creativity, or change. It is not difficult to see how crucial these factors are in learning. The unfamiliarity of the "Beware Agapanthus" sign forces a re-evaluation of habitual responses. We are forced to question and consider, or if the challenge is too extreme, we avoid. It is an important skill to "know what to do, when we do not know" (Claxton, 2003, p. 2), and it is something that is easily overlooked when there are so many prescriptive aspects of compulsory education.

My work setting

I now work as a creative practitioner/artist for a variety of museums, galleries, and schools. When I undertook the Psychoanalytic Observation Studies course, I presented some voluntary work as an artist in a primary school in work discussion seminars. The observational approach to this work and the reflection offered in the seminars helped me to refine my practice so much that I developed a career delivering creative projects.

In recent times creative practitioners/artists working in state education for national organizations like Creative Partnerships are being encouraged to formally adopt rudimentary forms of observation and reflection as part of professional practice. This has given a professional legitimacy to practices that I had developed but that were, until recently, perceived to be well beyond the role of an artist working in schools. The collaborative Action Research process promoted through Creative Partnerships involves developing a research question or hypothesis about creative teaching and learning and then using observation as a way of gathering evidence to reflect upon the question posed. This process involves creative practitioners and teachers genuinely working together and sharing a broad range of experience. The practical effect of this kind of Action Research is that both sides of the partnership are able to see that observation helps to develop good planning and delivery of projects, and that reflection and evaluation completes the professional development cycle. When this partnership works effectively, a confident creative fluidity emerges. Both practitioners are drawn away from familiar working practices towards unfamiliar ones. The Action Research process, which requires an evaluative document as an end product, pushes both teacher and creative practitioner to examine what "actually" happened and how best to collaborate in the future.

The delivery of the project reported on here was a collaboration between myself and a Special Educational Needs Co-ordinator with a Year 3 class and some children from an attached learning development centre. I had worked with the whole school over two days on one prior occasion before this project started, so there was some expectation from the staff and children that they would be involved in a different kind of learning experience. The project took place one day a week for ten weeks.

The Object Dialogue Boxes

I have made and developed a range of Bizarre Artefacts that are housed in boxes called Object Dialogue Boxes. The four boxes in existence each contain around 20 Bizarre Artefacts. The aims of the boxes are to stimulate creative thinking and dialogue and to act as catalysts for sculpture or creative writing.

The artefacts in the box under consideration here are modified "everyday" items housed inside a stripped, wooden cello case (see Figure 5.1). Often one object is merged with another object to create a kind of hybrid through which our conventional visual readings of the two original objects are thwarted. For example, one box contains a pair of second-hand shoe brushes that have had leather soles and heels added to the side of the brush opposite the bristles. When a participant picks them up and begins to think what the held object is, there is a mental and emotional fluctuation between an idea of a "pair of shoes" and an idea of a "pair of shoe brushes". A similar thinking process happens with the teapot pictured in Figure 5.2. Two disparate elements are linked by a coincidence in size: the teapot fits in the frame of the globe. The combination makes the teapot take on more "globeness", and the idea of a globe is stretched just far enough so that a "teapot—globe" is believable. Aesthetic intrigue and curiosity is stimulated. Consideration of what has happened to these everyday things asks us to look and think again.

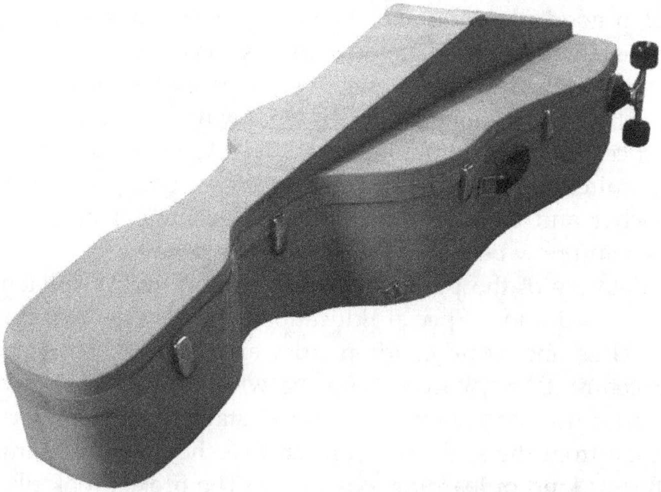

Figure 5.1. Object Dialogue Box.

I was interested in how handling and talking about such artefacts supports the development of young children's narrative skills. I suspected that one reason for the success of the project lay in the emotional impact of the artefacts on the learner. I think that the artefacts give a sense of authentic purpose, a real learning challenge that has to be overcome. There was a distinct pattern of engagement with the artefacts. The learners were presented with a small emotional chal-

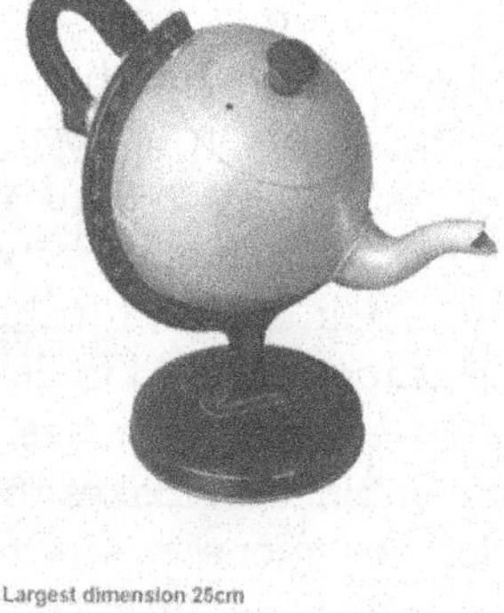

Figure 5.2. Bizarre Artefact: teapot on globe stand.

lenge, and the struggle to overcome this challenge was handled in different ways.

This approach has its roots in Lev Vygotsky's thinking about learning and promotes learning that is against the "transmissionary" model of acquiring knowledge, that is against didacticism and promotes, instead, a kind of co-inquiry between the learner and the teacher (Wells, 2000). Wells describes the process in simple terms: "To be able honestly to say, in response to a student's question, 'I don't know. How could we find out?' is probably more important, in creating an ethos of collaborative inquiry in the classroom, than always being able to supply a ready-made answer (Wells, 2000, p. 65).

This educational perspective is similar in many ways to psychoanalytic thinkers who have written about the subject. Bion "discriminates between a form of 'learning from experience', that changes the learner, and 'learning something' that might increase information, but does not change the individual" (Lopez-Corvo, 2003, p. 163). The key seems to be the relationship between teacher and learner. This is essential to establishing a genuine learning dialogue where the learner can internalize a dynamic and sensitive thinker. The mental space for this dialogue is the space Vygotsky referred to as the "Zone of Proximal Development". Reflecting on the Proximal Zone from a psychoanalyst's perspective, Friedman wrote:

> it is not necessary for the analyst to know the exact nature of the development he is encouraging. It is sufficient that he treats the patient as though he was roughly the person he is about to become. The patient will explore being treated that way, and fill in the personal details. [Friedman, 1982, p. 12]

In starting the learning journey with the Object Dialogue Box, the most important things are that the learning challenge is not too great for the capabilities of the children and that they are allowed the space to fill in the details. I visualize the Zone of Proximal Development as a geographical entity, a view of a landscape: where the children are standing is where their learning has reached, and their view to the horizon is the "Proximal Zone". The learner's perspective of the horizon depends upon whether they move towards it or, metaphorically speaking, how tall they are. Extending the metaphor, the learner can be helped to see more by standing on the shoulders of "more capable peers" and by being encouraged to move independently. To do this effectively involves the "more capable peers" calibrating the learning so that the learners are able to gravitate generally towards their own respective horizons without being pushed too much.

Introducing the Object Dialogue Box to the children

The children have completed morning registration and are sitting on a rectangle of carpet in one corner of the classroom. I introduce myself and explain to the children that they are going to be doing something very different from usual. I ask the class if they know what imagination is. The general consensus within the group is that imagination is something that we use in our heads to make things up, like stories or pictures. The class teacher has told the children that the project will involve writing and art (they have already written a baseline story inspired by a conventional object). I, as usual, have a degree of anxiety about whether the box will work; I recognize the feeling and remind myself that I have to sit with it.

I introduce the box and ask the children what they think it is. Anna says, "Violin, it looks like a violin shape." The children all seem to be listening and thinking; a few have put up their hands. Rebecca says, "It's a bass." I reply that that's an interesting guess. I want to congratulate the children for identifying it as an instrument case but wait to see what else emerges from their thinking. Richard puts his hand up eagerly, stretching as high as he can to be seen and to be picked to answer the question. "It's an E.T. case, it's got E.T. in it (Alien)." My waiting has paid off: we have moved quickly from what the object really is to what it could be. I congratulate the class. Paul gives me his idea: "A train . . . a little bit of a train . . . the carriage." There is complete concentration at this point. Tony tells me it is a mummy case . . . when mummies are dead because they get put in these kind of coffins. I reply, "Good, can anyone think of the word we use?" Tony has found the word: "Sarcophagus", he says with pride. The children are becoming more confident. Richard puts his hand up to ask me, "Could it be a monster—a funny-shaped monster?" I reply, "Yes it could be a funny-shaped monster." He continues, "It could also be a skateboard park, this bit (a raised section that houses the bow for the instrument) could be a ramp." John has a different opinion about the "ramp" of the case: "It could be a mini racing car because this bit is like that triangle bit that

> goes just behind the head (referring to the aerodynamic shaping behind the head of racing-car drivers)." Richard puts his hand up again. He has discarded his idea about skateboards: "It's a funny-shaped motorbike; you sit on the seat with the handlebars going that way." I reply, "Yes, it could be, well done." Tony has obviously been developing his own theme: "The Nile, it could be filled up with some water of the Nile."

The children do what one would expect and try to link the Object Dialogue Box to familiar concepts. They are familiar with the concept of "instrument case" but have not formed the concept "cello case" or perhaps even the concept of "cello". Other concepts of musical "caseness", such as "violin", are referred to by their instrument and are tried as approximates. I think "bass" is obviously intended as reference to a "double-bass case". However, the children have been made aware that this experience is in a different category of learning experiences and that we are looking for imaginative comments; perhaps this is a "sub-class" of the "super-class" of learning experiences. I feel that the children are aware a new class or concept must be formed and look for cues from myself to see if their attempts are valuable.

The desire to know

In the development of the Object Dialogue Boxes the starting point was the Bizarre Artefacts and their impact, but I found that if the learner could see all the artefacts at once, the sense of mystery, intrigue, and the "unknown" factor was easily lost. Putting the artefacts in slightly unusual boxes seems to activate curiosity and the inclination to create stories. It is this curious interest that brings to mind Melanie Klein's observations of the epistemophilic instinct at work within young children (Klein, 1928).

The anthropomorphic form of the cello case and its unfamiliar nature attracts a response. It could, perhaps, be described as "supervalent" for curiosity and imaginative inquiry. It is interesting to note that in the observation Tony imagines the cello case as *"a mummy case . . . when mummies are dead because they get put in these kind of coffins."* Tony is taking the anthropomorphic nature of the cello case and linking it to a subject that he has covered in the National Curriculum: he is being both creative and imaginative with what he knows and is familiar with.

Using a Bizarre Artefact

The following observation is a continuation of the session described earlier. The dialogue presented is intended to give the reader a sense of how the narrative emerges from the open questions that are posed to the children.

The Object Dialogue Box is still on the floor, and the children are sitting around it in an arc in front of me. I have their complete attention.

> I praise the children for their imaginative comments. I tell them that when we are using the Object Dialogue Box, whatever they think and say is fine, as long as it is not rude or offensive. I remind them that what they have just done is imagine what the box is and what its contents might be. I explain that the box is a cello case and ask them if they really think a cello is inside. There are mixed reactions. I delve into the box, keeping the lid closed as much as possible, and something starts to make a chirping sound. It is the teapot pictured in Figure 5.2, but without the globe stand. The teapot has a sensor inside so that when it detects loud noise, it plays the sound of a bird chirping a song.
>
> When I pull the teapot from the case, there is a mixture of stunned silence and raucous laughter from the children. As they begin to think about the object, they sit up on their heels, many with wide-eyed expressions. I ask the children what they think the object might be. Matthew puts his hand up to tell me that, "It's a teapot wot do this (dance-actions)." The other children laugh. Tony gives quite a literal explanation: he knows the real object that I have taken the sensor from. "A bird. I've got a Christmas bird like that." Some of the children begin to describe this toy. I do not deny or agree with them, instead I say: "Can we use our imaginations and say what it could be?"
>
> Suzie is the first to put her hand up; she says, "A mouse." I reply, "Yes, it could be a squeaky mouse." Richard says, "That could be the sort of blue thing with a hat in Aladdin." I realize that he means "Genie." I agree and then add, "What would this genie look like?" Paul responds quickly, "Like you . . . [meaning myself], a little bit smaller." Anna said, "It is a bird." This statement throws me a little: I feel as though I had been taken back to the conversation about the Christmas bird. Being sensitive to her contribution,

> I reply, "Yes it could be a bird." This comment had also thrown Richard off his thought; he reverts to trying to explain it, "You could have put a little bit of music in there but turned the volume down so it sounds like birds." I decided to try to get the process back on an imaginative footing. "Do you think that is more interesting than having a mouse or a giant's knee in there?" Richard says that he prefers imagining things and adds, "Could there be a little dinosaur in there?" I agreed with him, and another child says, "A dinosaur getting boiled." Somebody else adds, "It could be a Lion inside there." I like the association and look at the teapot as I hold it up. I put my ear to the Teapot and say, "What has happened to the Lion's voice?" Matthew puts his hand up and says, "The Lion ate a mouse that's trying to get out of his tummy." All the children laugh at this.

When the teapot had this sensor inside it, it presented the learner with a good introduction to Bizarre Artefacts. It is easy for the learner to know the teapot and know the sound of a bird; one might hear a bird singing while making a pot of tea. They coexist as separate categories or concepts—a sound that has no physical limits and a physical object. Symbolically, the sound represents the presence of a bird. The teapot is much more complex in symbolic terms; for the unconscious mind it might draw primitive projections based upon its container aspect, or the phallic nature of the spout. With less primitive projections, the focus might be on the symbolic associations linked to tea-making. The unknown quality that activates projection and nudges one away from the concept of a functional object that holds tea comes from a merging of categories or concepts. The bird song that comes from inside the teapot is a mixing of metaphors: we simultaneously "know" and "do not know" the experience presented to us. Bizarre Artefacts explicitly reverse the process of differentiation from which symbols can develop.

When this object was introduced, there was a mixture of stunned silence and laughter. I think that the laughter comes when the experience is recognized as symbolic rather than real, and this is the beginning of a form of play with the "shadows of imagination" (Coleridge, 1817). The struggle to link the artefact to an existing concept might be why Tony links the bird-sound to the Christmas toy, rather than playing with the idea. If the category of learning that we were engaged in was more readily identified as play, playing with our imaginations, then the process might stimulate less fear.

Writing stories

The aim of developing the Object Dialogue Box and the Bizarre Artefacts is to create a mental state of flux, a state conducive to creative thinking and inquiry. This process has a value in its own right, and children, or learners in general, should be the ones who find appropriate use for this. However, because of repeated pressure from learning organizations to deliver a product for this process, I have been obliged to demonstrate how it might help to deliver products relevant to the National Curriculum. The following passage will show how the Box can be used to help children create written stories that can be used as evidence of learning in literacy.

Session 4

In discussions the previous week (Session 3), the children had constructed a narrative around a bicycle seat covered in icing and cake decoration (Figure 5.3). We had been exploring character description and had come up with a character called "Ashley John". An indication of how the narrative emerges from the children can be seen in the following observations taken from the classroom. The key to the process is in forming open questions, such as, "Who might have owned this object?" Subsequent questions are aimed at amplifying what the children offer. It feels like sketching with words. The difficulty lies in tuning in to the narrative as it emerges. In the harmonization of the sketched elements disbelief is suspended, and more children become carried along in the process. I think that this is a less rarefied form of "reverie" (Bion, 1962a) that one might link to the "effective attunement" (Stern, 1998b) between mother and infant or analyst and patient. On many occasions I have found myself absolutely "lost" in concentration. This is also in part because I very rarely have the

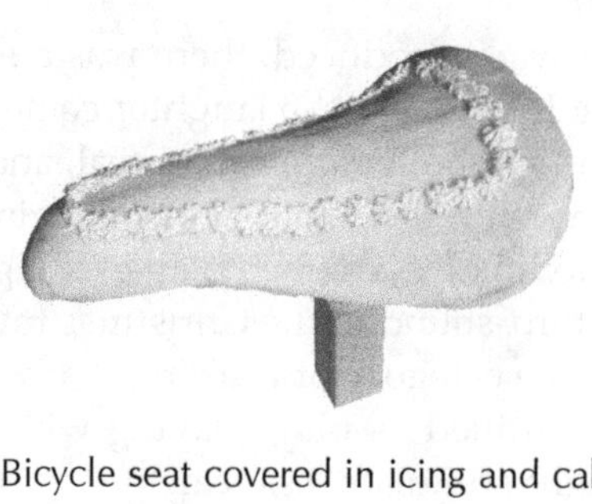

Figure 5.3. Bicycle seat covered in icing and cake decoration

luxury of a scribe and have to recap all that has been said. In this session Miss Sutcliffe had noted all the children's character descriptions on a flip chart. Later the roles were reversed, and I became the scribe for Miss Sutcliffe.

The notes that Miss Sutcliffe had made had been passed on to an illustrator so that the words could be translated into images of what Ashley John looked like. The illustrations were drawn on a large piece of card. The general idea of this learning process is that as the children co-construct a story, they will gain experience to help them do it for themselves. Over the next two sessions of the project the class will continue to shape the story around the illustrations and evolve it using new Bizarre Artefacts that I introduce. The story will be typed, the illustrations inserted into the text, and the text bound and distributed to the children to take home. Miss Sutcliffe, who has already begun to ascribe voices to the characters, will make a recording of herself reading the story so that the children who cannot yet read can revisit it at home.

> Morning registration is complete; all the children are sitting on the carpet, having given me a recap of the work done in the last session. We have discussed what illustration is, and I am standing in front of the children with the board (see Figure 5.4) facing away from them. When I turn the board around, there is a lot of laughter. A boy points to the top illustration and calls out, "That's him, that's Ashley John!" Miss Sutcliffe says, "Well, it might not

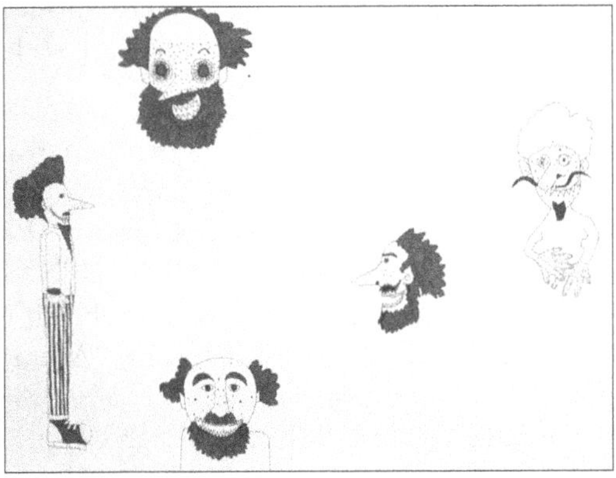

Figure 5.4. Ashley John.

be, other children might think it is one of the other pictures." Miss Sutcliffe sighs as Matthew starts to shout out which illustration he likes. She says, "Ok, Matthew, calm down!" I mention their earlier recollections from last week: "Here are his diagonal pointy teeth, and here is something that you didn't remember earlier, his moustache." One child calls out, "Oh, yeah", and I continue, "A pointy beard, big nostrils, spots all over his face, hairy hands, star eyes, and, as you wanted, he is very tall."

The children are asked to stand to vote for the various pictures. They choose the illustration that has a body. To check that they are not just voting for a "complete" image of a person, I ask them what they like about it. Alan puts his hand up, and Miss Sutcliffe asks him to explain. Alan says, "I am voting because I like the nose . . . and the teeth and the hands." Ronnie says, "I like his pointy teeth and his big bushy hair." Other children begin to talk over him, and Miss Sutcliffe gives a big "Ssssssh!" I explain that the illustrator might be able to make the odd correction if we have missed something out. I recap the children's descriptions, pointing to the words on the flip chart as I read them out: "Ashley John is 23 years old; he has bushy eyebrows. . . . The picture you have chosen does not have bushy eyebrows. Do you want bushy eyebrows?" Everyone shouts an enthusiastic, "Yeah!" I continue, "Oh, I have just noticed that you wanted spots all over his face, and the illustrator has just put them on his nose; do you want spots all over his face?" Jemma replies, "They are freckles!" Miss Sutcliffe looks at the flipchart and says, "Well, last week we wrote down that he had spots, not freckles." Ronnie adds, "They look like chicken pox." I reply, "Yes, they could be, but last week we agreed that he had spots all over his white skin, so I think that we should stick to that now."

Next, I take out the fencing mask (Figure 5.5) from the Object Dialogue Box. Ronnie puts up his hand and says, "What is it?" I am unwilling to answer at this stage, so I reply, "I am just going to ask the class this, so maybe you will be able to tell *me*? Ok, everyone, I wonder if somebody could say what it is?" Ronnie is excited, "A motorcycle hat!" Brian chips in, "A hat." Lucy adds, "A rugby helmet." Melinda says quietly, "I think it is one of those hats where you play sword fighting." Both Miss Sutcliffe and I give out gasps of amazement and ask what the name of the sport

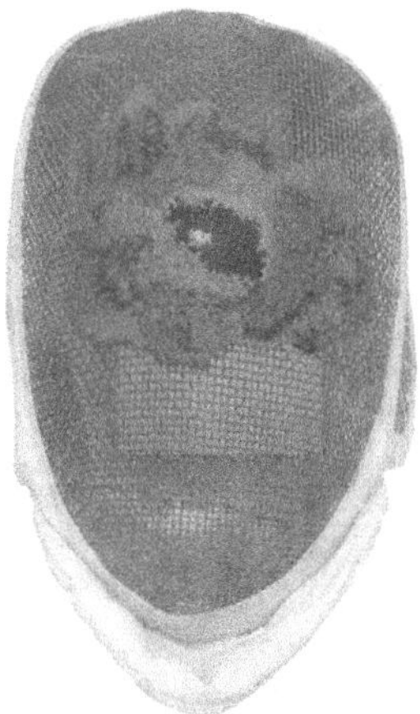

Figure 5.5. Fencing mask.

is. Paul has been sitting very quietly at the back. He puts his hand up, so I say, "Yes, Paul?" He replies, "Is it judo?" I tell him that it is not for judo, and Susan offers, "Is it a bees' hat?" I reply that it does look like a bee-keeper's hat. Wanting to shift the dialogue towards what it could be, I say, "In your imaginations it could be a beekeeper's hat, but in reality it is a fencing mask." I give a very basic description of fencing and try to move on, but Lee has not finished thinking this through. He asks, "Are they real swords?" Miss Sutcliffe intervenes, "No, but they can hurt you." I say they are blunt swords, but people need to wear protective clothing for fencing. Ronnie is sharply focused, "What do you mean, blunt?" To explain this, I pick up a sharp pencil that is in front of me and make an extended scribble on a piece of paper, leaving little lead left in the pencil. I say to Ronnie, "This pencil is a bit more blunt than it was a moment ago." A number of children nod with approval.

Moving on, I say, "Ok, that is what it is, but it has been changed a little bit. One of the questions I would like you to answer is: Is it old, or is it new?" Matthew replies, "Old." I ask, "How do you know it is old?" Matthew replies, "because it looks like it used to be white and now it is brown." I reply, "Good, there is a

> word beginning with 's' that describes the marks that are on it." No answer comes from the children, so I say, "When you spill something on a tablecloth, it leaves something on them if it is not washed soon after." Matthew calls out, "stains". I tell him that that was a good answer. I continue, "It has some letters written on the back of it. Can you see what it says?" The children peer forward as I hold it out for them to see. Somebody at the front says, "G . . . M." I then ask, "Why do people put letters on things?" Lee replies, "someone's initials?" I give him a big, "Yes!" in response and add, "You are doing well today." I continue, "The owner has put their name on it. Who could G. M. be? Does the mask belong to Ashley John?" I realize that I am asking too many questions, so I wait. Ronnie says, "The Magical Man." I agree.
>
> Miss Sutcliffe picks up the dialogue here: "If these are the magical man's initials, what could his name be?" A girl calls out, "Magical man." Looking flattened by this, Miss Sutcliffe tries again, "Ok, what could the first name be, something magical?" Somebody says, "George." I feel that this is ok, but Miss Sutcliffe continues to probe, and ideas start to emerge, "Grey Magician", "Green Magician", "Grotty Magician", "God Magician", "Growing Magician." Everybody in the class begins to get excited again. We take a vote, and the mask belongs to "The Growing Magician."
>
> To get a description of the "Growing Magician", Miss Sutcliffe and I follow a similar process to the one we used to develop an image of "Ashley John" (Figure 5.6). The children continue to use the fencing mask as an important object in the emerging narrative (Figure 5.7).

Eventually the children were given a complete illustrated version of the story that emerged, entitled "The Apple and the Sawdust". The Head read out the story at the school assembly, with the illustrations projected onto the walls. The children were thrilled and were offered the option of making a bound, illustrated book of their story. This offer added further impetus to the development of the children's individual writing. Knowing that their best stories would be submitted to an editorial panel for selection in a bound book gave them a sense of authentic purpose. Dramatic progress was seen in the writing of the majority of the mainstream children. Many children were dis-

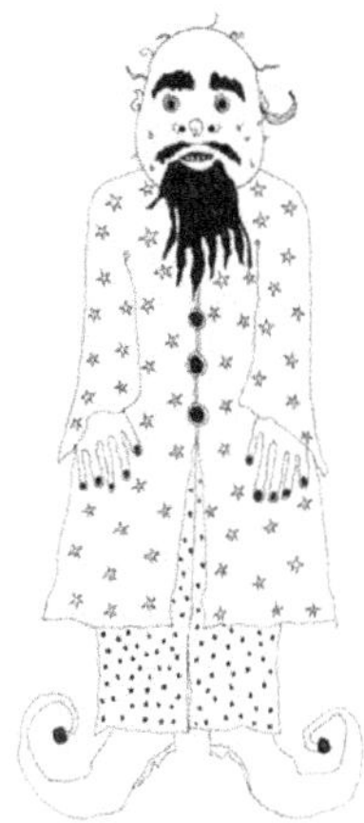

Figure 5.6. The Growing Magician.

appointed to stop writing at lunchtime, and some took work home to complete. The discussions about the Bizarre Artefacts became much more fluid and colourful, and the presentation of new artefacts was met with eager anticipation.

Writing analysis

I will give some evidence of the kind of development that took place by looking at the project teacher's analysis of the ten stories the children created over the ten weeks. I have selected Ronnie because his

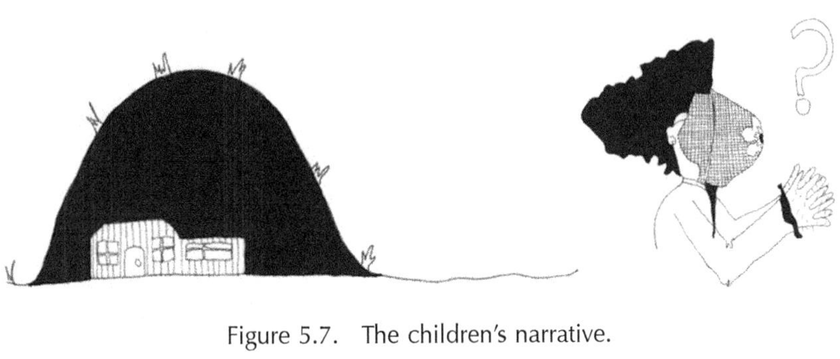

Figure 5.7. The children's narrative.

writing improved, and there was a distinct shift in the quality of what he was writing.

Ronnie, Year 3

Ronnie involved himself in the class discussion from the beginning, but many of his ideas were derived from books or videos. For the baseline task, Ronnie was given a very round pebble.

Ronnie's first story using a Bizarre Artefact from the dialogue box (silver goblets with pencils attached inside as kind of bell-ringers) was called "The Magic Trophy". He used the theme of "The Sword in the Stone" and adapted it to fit in with the objects. He began "*Once upon a time*", and it was about a boy who needs a trophy to become king. He introduced a new character into the story: "*a huge charanchaler*" (tarantula).

By Week 6, Ronnie began to use different openings: "*One sunny morning*"; "*Sam the tiger was angry.*" He also began to name his characters. The story was still action led with little description, but the sequence of events was thought out. He still relied on a familiar ending.

In Ronnie's final story he displayed confidence in using his own original ideas. His use of vocabulary was more imaginative, and he did not feel the need to move the action on so quickly. The story, "Africa's Party Day", begins:

"*It was the hottest day of the year in the land of Green.*" This opening sentence draws the reader into a sultry and unknown landscape. "*They disappeared all the way to a wooden hut. . . . Tango and Jamie opened the wooden hut door. There were thousands of African men and women dancing and singing. The African men and women dragged them in. Then they all danced and sang.*"

The language allows the reader not only to see the scene, but also hear the music and experience the atmosphere. It would seem that Ronnie is beginning to realize that a written narrative does not have to be all action to engage the imagination of the reader.

The most noticeable change was in the way he started to use idiosyncratic symbols instead of borrowed facts from existing stories.

> To use Bion's (1962a) understanding, Ronnie's learning and communication seems to be based upon his own experiences rather than learning and communicating "about something".

This finding was quite commonplace and seemed independent of children's ability.

Defences

The fencing mask in the last observation from the classroom delivers quite an aesthetic and emotional "punch". Adults and children alike are intrigued, and sometimes adults are fearful of it. The symbols that are hyphenated—"fencing mask–poppy"—constellate thinking in quite different ways, depending upon whether an adult or a child is discussing it. Adult dialogue around this artefact usually forms narratives in which it is commemorative in some way. Many adults see fencing as a kind of staged conflict, or play-conflict, and the associations around poppies as symbols of remembrance combines to create the commemorative dialogue.

It seems that children read the symbolic communication from Bizarre Artefacts differently from adults. If the work of art contains an array of symbolic communications, a mixture of primitive concrete symbols, symbolic equations, and symbols proper, they will read at the developmental level they have reached. The children use the mask in the narrative for its transformative powers; even though poppies and commemoration were discussed, these narratives were left out of the story. The children inquire about the protective aspects—the "beekeeper's mask" protecting from bees, and how other types of clothes are needed to protect the body from the swords. On reflection, my blunting of the pencil as a demonstration of what the term "blunt" means might have diminished the anxiety about the conflict under discussion. This is a symbolic discussion about the violent (pretended and made safe through a sport) attempts at penetration of another's body and how to defend against it. The "punch" of the Bizarre Artefact needs proportionate emotional strength to withstand it.

For the children the fencing-mask has wish-fulfilling powers like the teapot with the genie inside it: placing it on the head activates them. In the story that the group of children create there is a "conflict" over the mask between the "Growing Magician" and "Ashley John".

Having given the fencing mask to Ashley John out of generosity, the Growing Magician repossesses the mask and its powers by stealing it back. The conflict is resolved in Ashley John's favour because he suddenly throws another object at the magician, forcing him to drop the fencing-mask. I had introduced a new Bizarre Artefact for discussion at this stage: a 3-ft-wide balloon that had been filled with helium and was allowed to deflate over weeks. The effect of this object on the magician was that he, too, diminished in size and eventually disappeared. As a symbol one might associate an inflated balloon with hubris and a lack of grounding. At an unconscious level I may have given the children the deflated balloon as a diminishing symbol, the means of grounding the powers of omnipotence that had been located within the mask. In Ashley John's hands the fencing-mask had the feeling of a good psychoanalytic object; when the Growing Magician stole it back from him, the good object became dangerous. Good and bad co-exist within the fencing-mask; the danger comes from who is in control of it and what their impulses might be.

The key to the success of the projects with the Object Dialogue Box is that learning is negotiated. The "punch" of the Bizarre Artefacts presents a challenge in that they require adaptive learning. If the learner allows the emotional experience of the artefact to impinge, a change is generated in the organization of concepts and classes. The opportunity to work with the objects on their own allowed the children a private revisiting of the process. Each weekly session began with the types of discussion I have described. After a short break the children would choose to sit at a table on which was placed a Bizarre Artefact. The children could choose an artefact they had worked with before, or a new one. The children would write for 40 minutes, and then some of the stories would be read out in class. During the writing sessions erasers were not allowed, although crossing out and revision were positively encouraged.

As long as the form and pace of the dialogue is non-intrusive, change occurs in accordance with to the children's ability for it. At moments of excessive change, or poor containment, the symbolic process breaks down, as described by Money-Kyrle (1977).

When the writing of the children with significant learning difficulties was assessed and analysed, there was little improvement, but this belies the qualitative nature of the experience of working with these children. They became more able to contribute to the dialogue, and towards the end of the project two or three of these children told adults that they loved writing about the objects. At the beginning, these same children had been very reluctant to engage, even with the aid of a scribe. The following comments written at the end of the project are from the parents of these children:

> *"Rupert has taken to writing and drawing at home and making models without prompting and using his own initiative."*
>
> *"Tracey has been inspired to write stories at home which she never did before . . . for Tracey writing in workbooks is a chore, but this has made writing fun and something she wants to do. The project has also made her look at everyday objects in a new way . . . she can now see a face in her baked potato."*

Conclusion

The Object Dialogue Box and the Bizarre Artefacts present the learner with an aesthetic impact and an emotional challenge. Through the process of using them, habitual responses to new or unfamiliar experiences are challenged and explored. One of the first challenges for the children is how to negotiate a different type of learning, one that asks them to begin a kind of co-inquiry where there is no specific answer. Through this open inquiry the children become involved in learning that has a sense of authentic purpose.

The impact of the Object Dialogue Box and the Bizarre Artefacts is one of aesthetic conflict, a disturbance in the familiar harmony and beauty of the world, causing temporary disturbance to conceptual development. The key to their relevance is their emotional complexity. Children must be able to find some form of emotional correspondence within the Artefacts for them to be of relevance. Creating dialogue around the objects is a valuable process, because children internalize the experience of opening up mental space and allowing something to emerge.

The emotional punch delivered by the Bizarre Artefacts varies in its potency, but there is a degree of self-regulation through defences and existing patterns of behaviour that limit the impact. Some children disengaged by mentally opting out and others slow the pace of the dialogue or momentarily stop it. The Bizarre Artefacts seem to have enough inherent capacity to intrigue and then reengage the children when they can cope.

The project made a significant impact on the writing and narratives of most of the children from mainstream school. But the children did not see it as learning! Maybe they have acquired a new conceptual "sub-class" or "super-class" of learning experience. John's comment is representative of the feelings and thoughts of many of the children:

"I am sad it's over, because now we'll have to do proper work."

CHAPTER SIX

Work in health and residential settings

A Working with sick children in a hospital setting

Claudia Henry

This is an account of work I did as a hospital play specialist (HPS). I worked on a high-dependency 12-bedded surgical ward, which I shall call Badger ward. The problems the patients presented were mainly gastric, and there was a mixture of short- and long-stay patients. The children varied in age from neonates to 16 years old. I worked closely with the children, but also with their siblings and parents.

There was a playroom on the ward where much of my work took place. It was a safe area for the children, and I tried to ensure that no invasive procedures were performed on them in this room. I also worked with the children by their bedside when they were too unwell to come into the playroom.

In my role as a play specialist I had no specific structures to my day. Things on the ward were forever changing—children who seemed well enough to be in the playroom could, from one moment to the next, become very ill. There was an endless sense of vulnerability and anxiety, which I sometimes found overwhelming. I will focus on my battle to keep on thinking in spite of this anxiety and to keep on holding on to all the signs of life where there was often a real risk of death.

The beginning of my work with Carlo

My work with a child I will call Carlo was a formative experience for me: I present a narrative of the year that I spent working with him.

Carlo is the second child of Spanish parents. His sister is 12. He was admitted to the hospital when he was 2 days old with a serious bowel malformation. He was immediately operated on, and the bowel was found to be so damaged that it was all removed apart from 3 cm.

I met Carlo when he was 2 months old, when I started working on the ward. At the age of 4 months, he developed a mitral valve heart infection, and he nearly died. He was taken to intensive care for three weeks. During this time his intravenous medication leaked, and this resulted in his right hand being burnt. He consequently lost one of his fingers.

When he was 15 months old, he finally went home. I felt a great sense of joy at his going home but also a feeling of loss. I hope that I will be able to convey what was for me a very rich and intense experience with this child and his family.

> I was first introduced to Carlo and his parents, Mr and Mrs L, by Tessa, the ward sister. It was my second day there, and I remember Tessa telling me during "hand-over": "This one is going to be here a long time."
>
> My first memories of Carlo and his family are closed doors and a darkened room. I remember knocking at the closed door and feeling that I was invading the family's privacy when I went in. I was yet another person, and why would they want a play specialist? Their son was too young and too ill too play.
>
> I tried to introduce sensory lights and black-and-white books to Carlo, explaining to mother that small amounts of stimulation might be good for him. I remember a great sense of uselessness. How could what I provided be of help? Looking back now, I realize that for Mrs L entertaining the thought that Carlo could play meant entertaining the idea that he was alive and that he might stay alive. While he was still so ill, this may have felt too painful. Attempting to engage him in play often became something that felt too painful for me too.
>
> Although I felt that I was invading rather than helping, I continued to knock at the closed door every day and gradually came to

be welcomed in. I would stand on one side of Carlo's bed while Mrs L stood on the other, and we would both look at him and occasionally talk about him. One of the first things she said to me was, "He is so little, and he has had so much done to him already." Her English was not very fluent, and when she became distressed, it was often quite hard to understand her. However, my perception of her immense grief was very clear.

Carlo's condition started to improve. He started to enjoy toys and people talking to him, and slowly he started to vocalize. The sound of his babbling could often be heard as I walked past his room. This was a period of short-lived relief.

I set up a time every day when I would spend some time with Carlo while Mrs L had lunch and a break.

One of the practical issues that I found hard at the beginning of my time with Carlo were all the lines attached to him. I was frightened and unsure of how to pick him up. I remember never really being relaxed in holding this small, vulnerable baby who, in turn, never seemed able to relax in my arms. I wondered what projections of anxiety from adults must have entered Carlo's system, apart from what the lines were putting into him. I hope my awareness of my anxiety, my thinking about it, may have lessened what I projected.

Mr L started to come less and less to the hospital, as he was working, while Mrs L very rarely left the ward. It was clear that the family had very little support, and Mrs L was very often alone with Carlo. Menzies Lyth (1988) writes, with reference to children making long stays in hospital: "Relatives, friends and neighbours mobilize effective support at first, but their support is likely to diminish as the situation passes from the acute to the chronic" (Vol. 2, p. 137). This seemed to be the case with this family, and I wondered whether staying with the pain of such an uncertain future became too difficult for friends to endure.

Cardiac arrest

When Carlo was 4 months old, Mrs L started saying that something was not right with Carlo and that nobody was listening to her. As I stood on the other side of Carlo's cot, mother shook her head and said that she was worried, and "A mother knows these things."

I had started taking Carlo down to the "sensory room" during some of my sessions with him. He would sometimes relax for short periods in the darkened room, and I experienced short moments of painful but real contact with him.

I went down to the sensory room with him on this occasion, and it was clear that this time he could not settle.

> I held Carlo on my lap. He arched his back, and as his face turned to face mine, he looked directly into my eyes for a moment and then closed them and, bringing his hands in fists up to his face, started to cry. I took Carlo into my arms and rocked him, saying, "Hey, Carlo, it's OK, look, can you see the lights on the wall?" I was aware, however, of a sense of it not being all right. Carlo was hot, and his little body was jerky and tense. He did not seem able to find any comfort. I felt filled up by his distress. During this session I felt for the first time consciously scared at the responsibility of being away from the ward with him. I returned to the ward, and Mrs L seemed quite relieved that someone else had noted Carlo's acute discomfort. "I know there is something wrong", she kept saying, "and nobody will listen to me."
>
> Carlo had often fluctuated in his physical well-being, and I, although aware of Mrs L's worry, wondered if this would just pass, and he would be better again in a few days. I think at this point I was not only finding it hard to stay with Mrs L's anxiety, but I had also closed off a feeling of real fear and pain that had overwhelmed me when I was in the sensory room with Carlo.

When I came back to work next, I heard that Carlo had that very night had a cardiac arrest and was in the paediatric intensive care unit (PICU).

When this happened, I became aware for the first time of the sense of what can only be described as doom hanging over the ward. The laughter that I often heard from behind the nurses' station became at times quite hysterical, and I felt that we were all working through a foggy veil. What had happened to Carlo was hardly mentioned. This was to be a pattern that I started to recognize on the ward and one that would loom very large whenever a child died. Questions were asked by the ward sister in the same tone, it seemed to me, as if I were being asked if I would like a cup of tea. "Have you been down to PICU to see Carlo?" or "Are you going to Timothy's funeral?" The questions often came so suddenly and with so little feeling attached to them that I often found myself not able to answer. It became clear that in an environment where life and death are so close to one another, the feelings that surround and overwhelm one may not be acknowledged. Things would mechanically continue in the same vein but with heightened "humour" as a form of manic denial. Avoidance of the underlying anxieties often brought to my mind Isabel Menzies' paper on institutional defences against anxiety (1959). They seemed so clearly visible at times on the ward, and I was *not* immune to them.

It took me a few days to go down to PICU to see Carlo, and Mrs L. I became suddenly very busy, and each day would go home not having "had time" to go down. This pattern became clear to me, and I was aware of my own defence mechanisms and how easy it was to be "too busy". I was scared of having to see Mrs L's distress and pain. I was scared of having developed a relationship with this child who was now so ill.

When I did go down, I remember that Mrs L seemed almost not to recognize me at first. Her face was pale and full of pain. Carlo was lying sedated on a ventilator, and she was standing by his side looking at him. I stood as I had done on many occasions on the other side of the bed. There was silence, and then Mrs L said, "He can't play now." I had no answer. I realized, as the days passed, that my role during this time was just to listen and to hold some of the overwhelming and unbearable pain so that Mrs L could continue to care for Carlo. I had no answers, and I realized that I did not need them.

While Carlo was on PICU, his intravenous medication failed and burnt one of his hands. This resulted in his losing one of his fingers. I realized that confronted with the enormity of this suffering and what felt like such injustice, I started to back away again. I found visiting Carlo and Mrs L in PICU so distressing that I started to wonder if I was being any help at all. My feeling of being useless became more and more powerful and at times felt almost paralysing. I became acutely aware of the helper's need for help and realized how fortunate I was to have help from other sources. I often went home during this time overwhelmed and in pain and yet with a feeling of numbness that, with the help of my seminar group and analysis, I was gradually to start recognizing as my defence mechanism, my way of not feeling. I became aware of an intense wish to stay in the situation and fight against my internal withdrawal and not to get pulled into the coping mechanisms of the institution. Menzies Lyth writes about the need for defence mechanisms to stay in place being "greatest in institutions whose social defense mechanisms are dominated by primitive psychic defense mechanisms, those which have been collectively described by Melanie Klein as the paranoid-schizoid defenses (Klein, [1946], 1959)" (Menzies Lyth, 1988, p. 79). The feelings that I found myself confronted with during this time often felt very raw and provoked great anxiety within me.

To try to save Carlo's hand, leeches were used to help drain the blood. Mrs L kept on repeating over and over again in a low and profoundly sad voice, "Leeches—they are using leeches on his hand." It was as though the comparison between all the high-technology machines that were keeping Carlo alive and the savage simplicity of the leeches as a remedy was unbearable for her. I wondered what fantasies this blood-sucking creature was evoking in Mrs L.

Perhaps she felt in some way that Carlo's clinging to life, surviving when he shouldn't have, was in some way sucking the life out of her. She started to become very angry and desperately wanted to get Carlo back to Badger ward, away from the "blood-sucking pain" of the intensive care ward and the staff for whom she had developed a mistrust. Getting Carlo back onto Badger ward became her main concern, and in fact Carlo came back to the ward perhaps sooner than would be usual. This put a lot of pressure on the nurses, as Carlo still needed a great deal of attention.

The impact of the shock: "closing down"

When Carlo returned to Badger ward at the age of 5 months, he was a very different boy from the developing baby who had left. Very shortly after he returned, Mrs L started again repeating that she had known that something was wrong with Carlo and that nobody had listened to her. Mr and Mrs L's trust in the whole hospital was lessening. Mrs L would not leave Carlo's side and gradually became more angry and more depressed. She would walk around the ward crying, and Tessa, the sister, started to comment on the effect that this was having on other parents.

Carlo had become very withdrawn, and his only real response was to cry. He stopped using the right-hand side of his body—the side that had been burned—and he seemed to close down in a way that was not at all surprising, given the many painful invasive procedures he had endured.

He would not smile or vocalize, but he always watched, and I was aware of a very intense and alive eye contact. It felt that sometimes his stare was a persecuted one. He seemed to have become a child who had suffered what he must have perceived as so many "assaults" that his trust in others had disappeared. But I was also aware of elements of curiosity in his gaze. I believed that although he was not outwardly developing, he was still absorbing life into a hidden place within himself.

This period was probably one of the hardest for me. My belief in Carlo's hidden vitality felt very isolated and was very vulnerable within me. There were questions as to whether he had suffered neurological damage. It was sometimes easier to believe that this was the case. If I took at face value Carlo's closing off and lack of contact, then I could believe that he did not feel anything. I had to fight with myself to go on believing that it was the trauma of what he had suffered and not a neurological problem that was stopping Carlo from developing. Various neurological tests were done when the pain of Carlo's arrested development became too unbearable for those caring for him and an answer was sought, but all the test results were negative. Many of the nurses started to find it too "difficult" to look after Carlo. "His mother was too demanding and wanted his medication at exactly the right time." I would often try to share my view that this may be the only control that she felt she could exert, making sure her son got his medication at the right time. For many of the nurses the pain of Mrs L's anxiety and Carlo's suffering was too much, and of course they had other patients to attend to and couldn't always be there at exactly the expected time.

Mrs L was still positioning Carlo in his cot as though he were a newborn, and he spent most of his time lying on his back. She always seemed very sceptical at my suggestions of play. I wanted to find a way of installing some routine and normality in Carlo's life and to help Mrs L find a way of allowing Carlo to be alive.

I was aware of how scared she was and how fragile he must have seemed to her, and her heightened anxiety often overflowed into me. She would often show me his little hands covered in pinpricks from where blood had been taken and say, " It is too much, it is not fair." His hands covered in little pricks made me think of Esther Bick's paper on "The Experience of the Skin in Early Object Relations (1968). Perhaps Mrs L's ability to act as the "skin function" for Carlo's still unintegrated personality had been damaged by her experience. Mrs L was clearly so full of pain and anxiety, I often wondered what Carlo saw when he looked into her eyes. Was Carlo's "closing down" partly because of unobtainable catastrophic anxieties?

I sometimes wondered if I was too hopeful and not acknowledging the reality of the situation. Perhaps Carlo *was* too ill to play. In her paper "Helping Children Cope with Dying", Erna Furman (1984) writes about the need at times for the adult to stop asking the child to "eat, exercise, play, talk" and instead help them to "carry" the burden, which may mean a withdrawal from these areas that are to do with continuing life. With Carlo it always felt so unclear as to whether he was a "getting better" or a "dying" child.

Recovery: getting to work

Carlo's feeding had started to be nearly all through a tube. He would take by mouth only a special rice water that his mother would lovingly prepare.

One day, when Carlo was 9 months old, I was holding him on my lap.

> Mrs L came back into the room, having prepared his rice water, and started to feed him through a syringe. Carlo hungrily opened his mouth for the water, and I commented on the fact that he really seemed to like the food that she had made. Mrs L smiled and said that she gives him the water, and she eats the rice. She then said that Carlo has everything through a syringe: his medicine, his food, his injections.

The medical team were quite sceptical as to the good the rice water was doing. It seemed, however, that as an emotional exchange between Mrs L and Carlo it was to do with sustaining hope and life. In the seminar group we discussed the importance of Mrs L feeling that she could give Carlo something good, and the association between the rice water that Mrs L could make for her child and give to him as the closest she could get to breast-feeding. Carlo was, however, constantly vomiting, and as soon as the rice water had been swallowed, he would often bring it back up.

With the help of the seminar group I managed to keep the belief in Carlo's wish to live alive in myself and thus set up regular play sessions with him and joint sessions for him with myself and the physiotherapist. It felt at first that Carlo had lost the ability to distinguish between invasive touch and normal touch. He had previously needed physiotherapy on his hand, which had been very painful. He perceived Jane, the physiotherapist, as another person who inflicted pain on him. She, however, was adamant that she was not going to just hand him over to another physiotherapist. She was also aware of a liveliness somewhere behind all the pain, and we formed a mutually supportive partnership and kept on with the sessions.

Carlo would often cry in a terribly persecuted and painful way and would often vomit after having cried. It became clear that he was beginning to be able to make himself sick, perhaps as a way of evacuating all the frightened feelings of painful invasion he had had when he was touched. Although difficult to stay with, I felt that in Carlo's crying one could feel that he had not given up, and that this was a time and a space where he knew his cries would be heard.

Carlo had been classed as being in heart failure since his return from PICU, but as yet was not strong enough to have his mitral valve replaced. This provoked a high sense of anxiety for both me and Jane as we worked with him, as each time he cried his heartbeat would increase dramatically.

We persevered with the sessions, and after one occasion when Carlo was 10 months old and he had been so distressed that Jane had started to cry, a shift in Carlo's ability to interact came about.

This is an extract from that session.

> Carlo sat between Jane's legs, facing me. She said, "Look, Carlo, there is your friend." Carlo sat with his hands locked in fists raised above his head and for a while watched me. I showed him one of the squeaky toys and said, "Look, Carlo, this one feels soft." I helped him to feel the texture of the toy with his good hand, and he placed his hurt hand in his mouth, still in a fist." He then started to cry and arched his back, pushing himself backwards in order to lie down. Jane said firmly, "No, Carlo, you are not lying down, we are not doing anything bad to you." I picked up the bubbles. They have often helped to calm Carlo down. For a moment he stopped crying, but he still whimpered. I caught one of the bubbles on the end of the bubble wand and said, "Look, Carlo, can you pop it?" I showed him how it pops and said "Oh, where has the bubble gone?" Carlo watched, as he always does, but did not respond. His whimpers were now becoming more forceful cries, although there were no tears. I said, "Hey, look, Carlo, where are the bubbles?" We continued with this for a while, and I continued to catch them on the wand so that I could help him to feel them. There seemed to be two Carlos there—one who was crying and desperate and one who

> was actively engaged with the bubbles and me. Carlo, then, in the middle of his crying, for the first time reached out his hand and popped one of the bubbles that I had caught at the end of the wand. I felt such a sense of joy at his having achieved this and tried to show him by clapping and telling him how clever he was. Carlo continued to cry but was still completely engaged with the bubbles. After a short while he again reached out for another bubble.

His return to interacting while crying seemed to portray his internal struggle to find a belief again in life and living. If he reached out for something was it possible that nothing painful was going to happen to him? Could he cry and be angry for all that had happened and yet somewhere still have enough of a feeling of safety to start developing again?

It seemed significant that Carlo's first move towards something was to the bubble—something that is so precarious and vulnerable. Both for Carlo and for those working with him, his life felt so precarious.

Carlo started from this time to tentatively and slowly re-establish contact. Even his smile started off as a half-smile involving only one eye and a small part of his mouth. Mrs L commented at this point on how difficult it had been not getting any response from him and never knowing whether what she was doing was giving him any pleasure. "Maybe he was in too much pain to smile." I was aware of the joy, but also of a great feeling of pain evoked by Carlo's progress, as it did make clear how much discomfort he had suffered. Mrs L seemed during this time to become quite depressed. Carlo's life was still so vulnerable, maybe too vulnerable and uncertain for her to start really believing in a future for him and with him.

Linking up

Although Carlo was progressing developmentally, he was still having many physical setbacks and was constantly vomiting. As before, Mrs L started voicing her concerns about Carlo, and, as before, it felt that no one was really listening. The surgeons would often walk past Carlo's room without going in to see him. They, too, it felt, were not sure how to proceed with him. I could see Carlo's discomfort during our sessions and was very aware of Mrs L's feelings that her son was invisible to the surgeons. During a ward round, when once again

Carlo had been "overlooked", feelings of anxiety and anger became even more powerful in me. Rather impulsively and perhaps on Mrs L's behalf, I took Carlo in his pushchair and stood next to the group of surgeons and doctors until they looked at him. I explained that he was constantly being sick, that there had been blood in his vomit, and that he was clearly uncomfortable. One of the surgeons looked at him and said, "Oh he is fine." He was anything but fine, but was he at least strong enough for the heart surgery, the only procedure that might help him to stay alive? I felt helpless and useless. I was also aware that I had stepped out of my role.

Although the encounter with the surgeons had not helped, shortly after this an ethical review with all professionals involved was called to decide whether it was right to go ahead with the heart surgery to replace Carlo's mitral valve or, alternatively, to send him home on palliative care.

For me, the meeting was very difficult. The task seemed to be to decide whether Carlo should be allowed to carry on fighting or should be allowed to die. It was, however, the first time that all the people who were involved in Carlo's care had come together, the first time that he was being looked at as a whole child. It was unanimously decided that if Mr and Mrs L agreed, which I was sure they would, although there was a risk involved in the surgery, it should go ahead.

If the operation were to succeed, Mr and Mrs L could be taught the nursing skills they needed to continue giving Carlo his medication at home.

I remember this meeting evoking so many feelings in me: hope that there was a possible ending in sight to Carlo's hospitalization; thinking of my loss if and when he did go home; and anxiety about the possibility of him not surviving the operation. For the moment, Carlo's life still seemed to be based on so many If's.

Although anxious, Mrs L seemed relieved that some framework had been established and that somewhere in the distance there was a possibility that she could take her son home. I tried to stay with my new feelings of hope and focus on Carlo's ever-growing desire and fight to "wake up" from his long, painful sleep. He started to sit with no support, and his half-smiles became ever more full. Most importantly, it seemed that his capacity to attract people with his smile rather then to frighten them away with his pain was blossoming, and he started to see smiles rather than anxiety reflected in other people's faces.

Going home

Carlo had his operation when he was 11 months old. When I went to work after he had had it, the nurse in charge told me: "He is doing so well. He came off the ventilator the day after the operation and will be back with us tomorrow. He is our miracle baby."

Carlo came back to the ward, and Mr and Mrs L started their training to learn how to give him his medication and tube-feeding.

As Mrs L started to believe that her son was going to live and that she would be taking him home, I became aware that, for the first time, she started to buy him things. Up until this point all his toys, pushchair, and many of his clothes had been the hospital's. This reminded me of Romana Negri's writing about premature babies. She observed that while babies are still in a critical condition, mothers prefer to play songs and music that they liked to listen to during their pregnancy, showing that they feel the baby is still inside. As the baby gets better, they start to spontaneously buy toys that can be hung in the incubator. "The baby is no longer inside them; it is born and therefore needs a toy, the kind more suitable for a born child" (Negri, 1994, p. 29). While Carlo had been inside the hospital/womb that was keeping him alive, it may have been hard for Mrs L to really believe in his having been born and consequently having a future. Now that she could see an end to his hospitalization, he, too, needed objects suitable for outside the hospital/womb.

As the weeks passed and the time for Carlo to go home got closer, I became aware that the relationship between Carlo, his mother, and me was changing. Times that would have been play sessions with Carlo became very often times when Mrs L would hold Carlo and talk to me about her hopes and fears about going home and reliving some of the experiences they had had over the year. It was understandable and clear that there was still so much pain and a considerable amount of blame, which I tried not to encourage.

Holding Carlo as she spoke to me, Mrs L evoked a great feeling of loss in me. Both I and the hospital were handing the care of Carlo back to his mother. She was taking her son fully into her arms for the first time. My role had changed.

This is an extract from a session during this time.

> I sat on the floor in front of Carlo, who was in his pushchair. Mrs L was sitting on a chair on my right. It was five minutes past the end of my day. Mrs L had been telling me that if she had taken

> Carlo home when he was 4 months old, he would have been a nearly normal, healthy boy, but now she is taking home such an ill child. Mrs L, who is not usually physically demonstrative, then embraced both me and Carlo together in her arms and said, "Come on, Carlo, we have to let her go home now, we can't keep her here all night."

Mrs L must have had mixed feelings about taking Carlo home. Although she felt confident that she could hold him in her arms now, she was aware that she would be alone with him at home, with the full responsibility of his quite complicated care and the emotional impact of what they had been through. Although she wanted to go home, it still felt quite frightening. She must also have wanted someone to stay with her to help. Although I wanted him to be able to go home, I felt, as I said, a great sense of loss. Maybe this was why I stayed overtime.

My work with Carlo seemed to bring together many aspects of my role as a play specialist. One of the most crucial things I feel I learnt with Carlo was an awareness of the "closing down" impact of physical and mental pain, both on Carlo and on myself, and the importance of finding a way of keeping life and the thinking processes going through the pain.

On the day that Carlo left the hospital, he had seen countless people coming and saying goodbye. He had a strange expression on his face all day and seemed very aware of a change. As his mother wheeled his pushchair up the corridor on their way out, Carlo waved his new-found wave to everyone, and then, at the doors of the ward, he said the first clear word that I had heard him say: "Bye, bye."

B Trauma and containment in children's cancer treatment

Alison Hall

The aim of this chapter is to describe and discuss the dissonance between the ward nurse's role and the child's experience of treatment for childhood cancer.

Childhood cancer

"Cancer" is a generic term that covers both oncological (lumps) and haematological (blood) conditions. The incidence of childhood cancers in the United Kingdom is 1:600. The children can be grouped largely into two categories: high-dependency and low-dependency. The high-dependency children's treatment is typically more severe but of shorter duration (around seven months) and has a poorer prognosis than that of the low-dependency group, whose treatment lasts up to three years.

When treatment starts, most children quickly respond, and, as time goes by, their chance of relapse gradually diminishes, until after five years it is negligible—hence the term "five-year survival" equates to a "cure". The overall five-year survival rate is 65%. To attain a cure, the children undergo cyclical treatment with cytotoxic chemotherapy. Adjunctive surgery and radiotherapy may be required. The children have frequent general anaesthetics, bone marrow aspirations, and, at times, weekly lumbar punctures. Chemotherapy affects all cells, but healthy cells can regenerate while, hopefully, the tumour cells are killed off. While the healthy cells are recovering, and to cope with the side effects of the drugs, the child often requires supportive care. In a sense, after their initial stabilization, the children actually get sick *because* of the treatment we give them.

Setting

This work took place on the haematology/oncology ward on which I was a staff nurse. The children and adolescents on the unit range in age from new-born to 18 years old. For ease of referral, all will be referred to as "children". The unit has an average of 40 children in treatment at any one time. The ward team comprises 26 nurses, various support staff, and a multidisciplinary team within which there are six main doctors. The nurses work thirteen 12½-hour shifts per month. Other than the fact that one is never rostered on for more than three shifts in a row, there is no set shift pattern. On average, each nurse does one set of night shifts each month; thus there is no predictability as to when particular nurses might be on duty. During every shift the children are allocated to individual nurses. Though it is recognized practice to look after the same patients if you are on duty the following day, this does not always happen.

In writing about my work, I focus particularly upon two aspects of the child's treatment: the first is treatment that involves the piercing or entering of the skin, as this causes the most manifest distress for all involved; the second involves the post-chemotherapy phase, when the care the children require is due to the distress their own body causes them through side effects of the medication.

Despite material being available during every shift, I initially experienced great difficulty in achieving any consistency in the recording of observations. The variables in the ward setting are vast: diagnosis, prognosis, day shift, night shift, activity being observed, number and combination of people present, the child being observed. A review of the preliminary observations recorded revealed random and irregular accounts. I also realized that the preliminary material had been chosen to describe points that I wished to make, rather than allowing the material itself to present the themes. This highlighted Rustin's advice that

> It is important to this method . . . to keep the gathering of evidence and the making of theoretical inferences fairly distinct from one another. Theorizing at too early a stage . . . is more likely to be a

> defence against the pain of emotional experience or ignorance than a means of real understanding. [Rustin, 1989, p. 52]

The shift pattern ruled out a particular day of the week as "observation day", and, due to the unpredictability of admissions and subsequent care required, it was impossible to choose particular children or events. Hence I decided to choose the first shift of the week, for ten weeks, as my focus. The subject of the observation would be the child I was mainly involved with during that shift. I hoped that during the first shift of the week I would be less indoctrinated in institutional defences and more open to the situation I wished to record.

Two children are described. Each child features in an observation of what I call "external" trauma (the administration of painful treatments) and then "internal" trauma (when they are ill due to the side effects of the drugs).

External trauma

As part of their treatment, the children require many invasive procedures, and these are most frequent in the initial phase, before the staff are known to the child. No orifice is left untouched, and many new ones are made. In order to receive chemotherapy and the subsequent supportive care, the children all require a central "line" that gives direct access to their bloodstream. This can be either a Hickman line—a catheter that lies half outside the body, whose tip ends at the entrance to the heart—or a line that is similar internally but ends in a blind port, which sits under the skin of the chest wall. The latter—a "port-a-cath"—can be single or double and is accessed using a gripper needle. Ports are designed for intermittent use, and they are useful as, when they are not in use, the child can bathe and swim normally, and there is no "line" to be accidentally pulled or infected. The port can be mobile, so you must feel for it, then hold it steady before pushing the needle in (the skin can be numbed beforehand with a local anaesthetic). Gripper needles may stay in place for one week. Depending upon the port's mobility, its depth under the skin, and the skill of the nurse, it is possible for the needle to miss the port, which is the size of a thumbnail. This obviously adds to the child's apprehension and their requests that particular nurses do their grippers. Tasks such as gripper insertion are often the focus of nurses' skill acquisition—and observations showed that nurses' concentration at this time of learning often focused on the task and not on the child.

Though the chemotherapy the child receives does not vary between centres, the choice of lines does. In some centres all children get Hickmans, in others it is a family choice. In the centre where I worked, unless the children were high-dependency, they received a port. These differences are due to individual consultant and surgeon preference. The child's visit to hospital mainly commences with the accessing of their port—either for administration of their chemo or the supportive drugs (antibiotics, blood transfusions) required thereafter. Though the examples of external trauma chosen for the purposes of this chapter are of gripper needle and nasogastric tube insertions, the feelings that are described are applicable to other forms of external trauma. Procedures such as intramuscular injections provoked the same responses.

Observation 1: Ivy, 8 years old—gripper insertion

Ivy is an 8-year-old girl with a poor prognosis. Her family (mother, father, and 3-year-old sibling) home is a two-hour journey from the hospital. At the time of this observation, Ivy has been in isolation for three weeks undergoing a bone marrow transplant and is unwell, suffering the side effects of the high-dose chemotherapy. Prior to this she had already received a course of chemo via her port-a-cath every 10 days for 70 days, followed by a two-week rest, and then surgery to remove the shrunken tumour. For her transplant she had a double Hickman line inserted, as we could predict that she would require constant intravenous access, which would cause the skin over the port to break down. Today we require an extra intravenous access point, as Ivy needs to start a morphine infusion to control her pain, so her port-a-cath is to be accessed.

> . . . I kneel down beside her and say, "I'm going to do your grippers", and she nods, saying, "It's okay, 'cause you won't miss." I nod and say, "Remind me how you like this done", and she says, "Don't tell me when." I say, "Okay, I'll clean your skin first then get my fingers ready", and she nods.
>
> . . . I take the first gripper and Ivy looks at it and says with mild, but rising, panic, "I don't like them." Her Dad says, "We'll pad it up well", and I agree. I ask which port to do first, and she says the outer one. The fingers of my left hand hold her outer port steady, and my right hand has the gripper ready.

> Ivy says, "I'm not ready." I say, "Okay." She says, "I'll be ready in a minute", and I nod. I stay in position, as I remember that sometimes Ivy gets her confidence up suddenly, and once I missed that window of "readiness". . . . I keep quiet, as every so often her Dad asks if she is ready, and she replies, "nearly". . . . Maybe she senses I cannot wait for ages, as she says again, "I'm not ready"—looking me in the eye. I nod and say, "That's okay, Ivy, I will wait, but you need to try to get ready soon because Sue is waiting for her chemo." My arm is getting sore, holding the port steady, I say so, and that I am just going to give it a rest. She nods. I soon replace my fingers, and she says "Really nearly ready", and I sense she means it.
>
> She says "When I scream, put it in" and turns her head slightly towards her Dad and starts to scream. I push the needle in. I say, "It's in, Ivy", and she stops screaming and looks, taking some deep breaths, almost crying, and says, sounding relieved, "It's ages since I had them in, but that cream works." I ask if she wants me to carry straight on with the next one or have a break—she chooses a break.
>
> . . . I get ready for number two and she sees me, she turns her head to her Dad and, after only a few moments, starts to scream. I push the needle in, but just then she moves a touch or I do, and I need to push again, with conviction, for it to go in.

Due to past experience I was confident that Ivy would let me access her port and that I would get the grippers in first time. I felt Ivy's transferential panic when she saw the grippers, but it did not worry me. Perhaps in this way I contained some of her anxiety, calm in my countertransference. When she looked me in the eye as she repeated "I'm not ready", it felt like a challenge to see if I would—or could—share the experience of waiting and not take control and overrule her. On reflection, I see the waiting empowered Ivy to gain some control over the procedure that was taking place in the context of previous shared experience with me. Her scream is oppressive every time I hear it. Does it drown out all her other feelings in order for her to allow the piercing to take place? That the strategy she employed worked for her was evident in the speed with which she consented for the second gripper, and I was glad that, although I was not looking after her, we had agreed to her request that I insert her grippers.

Observation 2: Alex, 17 months old—insertion of nasogastric tube

Alex is the fourth of five children. He has a haematology condition with a very poor prognosis; at the time of this observation he had been in hospital for four months. Initially he had been very unwell indeed, but he is now quite well and is allowed out of the hospital today for the first time since diagnosis. His nasogastric tube requires replacing for the medication he receives six times per day.

> Alex is lying in his cot holding a whole Easter egg, half-unwrapped, up to his mouth, with smiling eyes. . . . I laugh and say, "Are you a happy boy." His Dad says, "well, I have to butter him up", gesturing towards the tube. As I prepare the tube, Alex is watching me. I say, "I have to put your tube back down, wee man." He immediately drops the egg and cries and looks to his Dad, turning his body towards his Dad's side of the cot. I ask his Dad if he is okay to hold him, or should I get another nurse. He says, "No, I'm fine." I get everything I need and go to the cot. Alex cries all the louder and tries to crawl up his Dad.
>
> Without speech, his Dad lays him down on his back, with one hand holding his arms across his chest as the other holds his head steady . . . I say, "Here we go, 1, 2, 3", and put the end of the tube to his right nostril. I keep on pushing until I feel resistance and stop for a minute. He continuously coughs and gags, his mouth opening wide, eyes shut; I worry that he will be sick. I continue to push the tube down. Once it has reached my marker, his Dad puts his finger on the tube at his nostril, obviously knowing the drill, while I get the tape on. We sit him forward, saying "It's in." He is pushing my hands away from him and still crying/complaining. I pull the guide wire out of the tube and withdraw some fluid with a syringe to check the tube is in his stomach (and not in his lungs).
>
> I begin to wash the guide wire, and Alex's crying escalates as he watches—he recognizes it. We both reassure him it's finished, and I move away. I go across the room to get his medications and return to put them down the newly passed tube. As I do so, he complains, pushing my hands away. His Dad is trying to make the tape stick, pushing it against his cheek, and Alex pushes his hand away and turns his face away. For the rest of the evening Alex ignores me every time I enter the room and

> protests whenever I do his temperature, and so on, by pulling away from my touch.

Alex immediately recognized the procedure that was to be done, and his reaction was instantaneous—the egg discarded, in his upset and panic to get into his Dad's arms. Though his Dad laid him on his back easily and he did not manage to struggle free, his distress and objection was desperate even before the physical procedure commenced. Despite our staff defences used in an effort not to relate, my deepening understanding of the child's experience was making invasive procedures more stressful for me. I felt myself clicking into preparation mode, impassively seeing Alex's panic but simply continuing on, without thought or speech. For neither adult to have spoken to him until the procedure was done seems unbelievable. For the rest of the shift I was aware of Alex pushing me away and protesting every time I went near him. I felt I had in some way betrayed his trust, as for a long time I had not been present during any painful events with him.

Internal trauma

Internal trauma occurs in the post-chemotherapy phase, when it is the child's own body that is causing distress due to the side effects of the chemotherapy. Here the nurse's role changes to one of carer and comforter, providing the supportive care the child requires to survive. There are many aspects of supportive care—intravenous and oral antibiotics and drugs, red cell and platelet transfusions, skin care, mouth care, pain relief.

Observation 3: Alex—general care

This observation took place two months prior to the insertion of the nasogastric tube. Alex was unwell, suffering from his disease, infection, and the side effects of chemotherapy.

> Alex is lying asleep on his belly, alone, when I enter the room. He has two infusions running through a femoral line in his right groin, a nasogastric tube, and a saturation probe on one toe. Dressings cover old line sites (the lines were lost to the infection) and he has a stitch from a recent biopsy on his flank. Much of his skin

> is raw and excoriated. He lies naked on a pressure relief mattress, to cool his temperature and to aid his skin healing.
>
> . . . I say, "I need to turn you, wee man, you are wet." He moans . . . he moans continuously as soon as I start to wash him and tries to hold my hands and pinch my skin. I spread some moisturizing cream on my hands to warm them. . . . His moans increase slightly, then almost immediately wane to a low "MMnnnnnnnnn" as I rub around his belly, then lift each leg in turn and "milk" it from ankle down to groin. He seems to enjoy this, closing his eyes.
>
> . . . He opens his eyes when his Mum comes in, and his moans get louder. He holds his arms out to her. She smiles at him and says, "Ali's creaming you up, my boy, thank you." As she walks around the room, Alex's eyes follow her. She is continuously talking to him; she comes over and says, "You want some booby, baby?" he nods, and she says, "Okay, then." His Mum leans over the cot, takes a breast out from her pyjama top, and offers it to Alex. He leans over and begins sucking it, making contented noises, with one hand under the breast and one on top of it.

His Mum and I then had a long talk about whether or not any of the siblings will be a match for Alex for a bone marrow transplant. Alex feeds throughout. . . . When I return to give him some IVs, he is alone.

> He is holding on to my glove, he slowly moves his fingers over the plastic. I look around for something to replace my hand (so I can finish his IVs) and see a balloon, and realize that is why he had liked having balloons in his cot—to hold on to. I put the tied knot in his fingers, in place of my hand; he holds on to it. He is moaning again, and so I sit and let him take my hand again, after removing my gloves. He is softly feeling it and occasionally gives it a nip. I ask if he is trying to hurt me, and he nods. I stroke his head, hoping he will nod off, and notice his heart rate dropping on the monitor as he does so.

I felt calm and competent caring for Alex, knowing I could make him feel better. I felt I understood his wish that I should not move or clean him, and when he pinched my hand, I felt I received his communication that it hurt (though it seemed advanced for his age when he agreed). While writing up the observation, I became very aware of his exposure and isolation and my hands in relation to him. It was heart-warming to observe a "normal" intimate moment between mother and baby breastfeeding and to realize that he could still draw upon such good experiences and hold on to them—as he did in finding a replacement object in my fingers, and in their absence, the balloon.

Observation 4: Ivy—general care

One week later, Ivy is no better. She continues on multiple antibiotics, anti-virals, intravenous feeding, and pain relief.

> I enter the room to give Ivy her drugs and read her infusions for midnight. The right side of her face is all crusty, red, and raw with shingles. She has two infusions running via her Hickman line, a morphine infusion via her port, and a gastrostomy tube connected to a feed. She has a saturation probe on her toe and an ice pack on her face to help with the shingles pain. One eye is swollen almost closed, and the white of the other is totally red from internal bleeding. Her abdomen is swollen but the rest of her body is skinny.
>
> . . . Ivy drowsily says, "What are you doing?" and I say, "I need your gastrotomy tube for your medicines." She lifts her T-shirt and says, "Is my feed off?" and I nod. She clamps her line, and I get the first syringe ready. Ivy queries the size of syringe and names the drugs I am giving her. She is trying to do them herself but is falling asleep, and I ask if I should do them; she says "okay" and sleeps through the rest.
>
> . . . I then put her IV fluids on hold and say, "I need to get your 3-way-tap for your antibiotics." "I'll do it." She lifts her shirt but is already falling asleep. Ivy says, "[the day nurse] was letting me do it myself", with her eyes half-shut (she is on a high dose of intravenous morphine—for which I had inserted her grippers). I say, "You can, if you wish", and she puts her hand over mine on the syringe and falls asleep. I push the antibiotic in slowly.
>
> I am just turning away when she sits bolts upright again, saying, "my bowl", and promptly begins to vomit. "Oh no, I've thrown my medicines up." . . . It takes a minute for the retching to calm down, and she is sitting cross-legged on the bed with her head down, bowl on her knee. She says, "It was the taste of that anti-

> biotic that made me sick, look at these tissues, they are nice" and rubs one on my arm. . . . I say, "Should I have done them the other way around? The IVs first and then the medicines." She says, "It wouldn't have made any difference." After some time she lies back down.
>
> . . . Again she suddenly sits bolt upright, saying, "I need the loo." There is a bedpan ready on the chair by her bed, and she gets up independently, guarding all her lines, and on to the pan. She says, "Oh no, diarrhoea again. . . ."
>
> . . . Later, I hear an alarm coming from her room. . . . Her nose is bleeding a bit, but by the time I am in the room (we must wash and put an apron on prior to entering, as she is in protective isolation) it is almost stopping. Ivy says, "It's just a little, I had platelets earlier anyway." She says she will sit up for a while. When I return, she is asleep in the chair, and I gently cover her with a blanket.

Ivy's apparent independence and ability to manage was at odds with the feelings her care aroused in me. I felt tired out in her room and could not imagine how she could be so active and independent in her circumstances, tied to five different machines and seven tubes. Her body seemed to be ravaging her, and yet she seemed resigned. Her switch from retching to nice tissues confused my feelings, and it amazed me that she could still gain such pleasure.

Discussion

External trauma

Bick (1968) describes skin as psychologically holding one together, creating a boundary between one's own being and others. When this boundary is constantly being pierced, as it must be in cancer treatment, there can be no sense of being intact, or even safe, in one's own skin. How does this feel for the child and for the nurse?

As Alex demonstrated, the children always seemed to be aware that a procedure was imminent, even if it was not discussed. A common theme for children of all ages was that they did not take these procedures passively. Their protest and alarm was evident in many ways: physically turning away, verbally shouting and pleading, silently ignoring you. Ivy was in the enviable position of comprehending why the procedure needed to be done and knowing that, this time, she could take control and procure the time to steel herself to consent. I know her ability stemmed from many previous hours of play preparation and our joint experience of such procedures.

Many children are not prepared, not given the time to get ready. Others are too young to understand why a procedure needs to be done, cannot consent, and have to be held down. It took me a long time to identify the stark reality of restraint as a theme, a fact that seems unbelievable now. However, these intrusive acts are not purely physical: there is an emotional reality to them as well. In examining numerous observations of painful procedures, I found that, in general, little nursing attention was paid to the child's communications. For this to persistently be the case, despite my deepening awareness, became increasingly painful and frustrating.

Most often, you don't know who put a child's grippers in, or how. On the unit it is not documented how a child likes a procedure to be done, and, more worryingly, seldom does anyone ask. Neither play preparation nor the play specialists are used consistently. Months earlier, when Ivy had been due her first gripper change, I deliberately did not offer to do it, so as not to impinge on another nurse's work and so that Ivy would not become "too reliant" on me. Thus, despite "knowing" that it would be better for Ivy if I did her grippers, the pressure not to defy the ward milieu had won. I regretted this decision immediately when I asked her nurse how it had gone, and I was told "Fine, I just whacked 'em in, didn't have time for a long thing." I felt frequent anger and frustration with my colleagues over such points, and the strength of these feelings exposed them as touching upon deeper issues.

Internal trauma

During internal trauma the child must literally trust us with its life, having previously, during external trauma, often fought against us. The repeated cycles of post-chemotherapy nausea, vomiting, and diarrhoea could be linked to infantile experiences of being fed, being sick, and defecating. Hopefully the child's experience as a baby will have been a healthy one, with good experiences outweighing bad, thereby assuaging some of the present unpleasantness. Alex certainly was able to make good use of his mother's "good" breast and even found a replacement for it in its absence, via both the balloon and my hand.

I realized that the children were so aware of their bodies and the physical space around them, it was almost as if their isolation cubicle was an extension of their body. Alex opened his eyes as soon as his Mum silently entered his cubicle. Ivy could name every medicine, knew when her lines were due to be changed and exactly what her blood counts were each day. It was her body that was now the enemy, launching surprise attacks.

My role during internal trauma seemed more caring. "Ill" children seemed to elicit more basic nursing care. Feeding, washing, observing bodily functions, monitoring, and measuring all input and output from the child's body are required; many of these actions make the child more comfortable and elicit gentler emotions. This would appear to be an "easier" role than that previously described.

Though in some of the care I documented I identified with the state of reverie that Lanyado (1985, p. 51) described as "sitting quietly at the bedside of somebody who is very ill and nursing them calmly and confidently back to health", as my work progressed I also found myself guiltily avoiding looking after the sickest children. This was unusual for me—normally I felt a sense of achievement knowing that good nursing care at this time can prevent deterioration and a trip to intensive care. I told myself "I couldn't be bothered" with "their IV workload", but I knew I did not want to face my growing awareness of the awfulness of the child's situation.

Pamela Smith (1992) wrote of the "emotional labour" required of nurses if they are to combat the stress arising from their work in ways that do not involve developing a thick defensive skin. A "thick skin" would ensure that patient communication bounces off, rather than being taken in, thought about, and responded to appropriately.

Staff institutional defences

The personal and institutional defences used within the health care system to combat the stress that this work invokes has been extensively described (Menzies Lyth, 1985; Robertson, 1958). Through thorough examination of the observations, many specific forms of staff and institutional defences became evident, ranging from the language employed by staff to physical equipment.

I found I was very consistent in explaining what I was going to do—for example, "Okay, I'll clean your skin first and then get my fingers ready"—but I realized that I did so in an almost ritualistic manner. This preparatory speech was used regardless of any communication from the child, and I began to wonder whether it was spoken as much to prepare me as to prepare the child. It seemed that once I was actually doing a procedure, my work-mode mind would often not respond to a child's questioning or protest—even though my observer's memory registered and recorded it. I would simply carry on informing them of the sequence of my actions, necessary for the task. Upon closer examination, I realized I also used language to minimize events. The word "just" featured innumerable times, "I'm just going to. . . ." I also did not use some significant words. Words that surely must describe how a child feels—fear, pain, and hurt—never featured in the observations.

As I wrote the observations, I experienced my hands looming larger than life and gloved hands appeared to be something to be feared: "As soon as she looked over and saw my gloves and tray, she started to cry" (Dee, 3½ year-old, intramuscular injection). I often say, "It's OK, I haven't got my gloves on yet." Once I am "gloved up", rather than having to start all over and don a clean pair, I would often wait for other people to do things (answer the phone, get the child). Gloves therefore appeared to have a dual purpose. They physically protect me (from chemo, blood products), and they form part of my psychological preparation and defence.

Another form of defence I began to recognize was the ability to "lose-in-mind" memories of certain procedures, which were dimly, but then vividly recalled later while typing up an observation. This ability to lose-in-mind must contribute to nurses' tendency as a group towards lack of communication, discontinuity, and fragmentation of knowledge. Hinshelwood and Skogstad (2002) describe nurses actively turning away from suffering. As time went by, I began to avoid certain procedures—and shun writing up observations. I felt I did not have the energy to write and could not access any reflection. It was as if I had begun to see a physical state, instead, a of child, as one sees a handicap when the person is unknown. It is distressing to examine one's own work and find it wanting, but these discoveries also reflect just how painful the treatment we must administer is. Both the individual and the system defend against open awareness.

The random distribution of shift allocation, and of who will perform a painful task, and how, for an individual child (overtly, in order that they do not become too dependent on particular members of staff) means that the child cannot predict who will be looking after him or her or anticipate how a procedure will be done. Menzies

Lyth (1985, p. 197) describes how the "number of staff is such as to risk multiple indiscriminate care-taking", echoing Robertson's (1958) research that associated indiscriminate care-giving with a denial of the meaning of children's communications. This system of working persists, used, albeit unconsciously, in order to protect staff. But is it justifiable? With such painful and intrusive treatment that lasts, in some cases, for years, should it not be mandatory that the emotional experience for both the child and the staff receives an equal amount of attention as the task?

Parents

For a long time, despite innumerable examinations of the observations, I was unable to access any substantial reflection or thoughts around parents in these situations—I felt they would require a separate observational focus. However, once I eventually acknowledged it, what was glaringly obvious was the fact of the parents' silence. In its absence, the very thing I was searching for became a presence—the presence of a lack of any displayed distress or protest: simply, the lack of speech. Judd (1995, p. 75) describes parents in this situation becoming "adamant, determined and rigid", detaching from the child's feelings in order to allow "torturous treatment" to take place. The parents face an awful dilemma—they want the treatment to take place in the hope that it will afford the child a cure—but they cannot want to see their child in pain. They seem to retreat to a state of silent assent.

During treatment, the parents' protective containment and the child's protective skin is constantly being pierced. When parents are present and compliant with painful treatment, the child must, at a basic level, feel that they have failed to protect them. Judd (1995) discusses parents' ability to act as a protective shield as depending on the extent to which they, too, feel traumatized. She replaces the word "shield" with "filter" in order to imply a two-way process between filtering that which is forced upon the child by medical personnel and the relaying of the child's responses back. I would argue that the filter can easily become blocked by the volume of painful procedures that the child with cancer must endure and the parent witness, leaving parents themselves simply trying to cope as the child's trust in them is continuously violated.

It must be very difficult to know that your child is ill because of the treatment you have consented to—while not knowing whether it will do any good; difficult, too, to require assistance to keep your child safe. The observations of internal trauma saw parents who were quietly present, containing, and comforting their children. The parent also has little control over the exposure their child has to the many different styles of care provided by individual nurses. It would be hard to complain, to risk being unpopular with the staff you rely on to care for your child.

Reflections

A haematology/oncology nurse's daily work oscillates between delivering the equally important invasive treatment previously described and caring for children through their subsequent illness. At some level there must be a concurrent feeling of omnipotence and guilt as potentially life-giving and certainly life-prolonging chemotherapy is administered. Such treatment might not always be in the child's best interests and subsequently makes them ill. The child, too, experiences this split: the same nurse who inflicts the external trauma later supports them when they are unwell.

The journey I have taken in documenting my work and the experience of children and parents, alongside an endeavour to understand the attendant emotions, was both a painful and an enlightening one. To realize just how active the children are throughout their treatment and to witness their ability to hold on to the good is very encouraging. Attending to the child's conscious and unconscious communications via observational skills assisted my understanding of both my own experience and the child's. Knowing that Alex liked to have a balloon in his cot came from nursing experience—but understanding why was directly linked to observational awareness. I also realized the strength of my anger towards my colleagues when care fell short of my standards (for example, when a previously compliant child was overruled or no play preparation performed). This emotion was probably no stronger that the strength of the nurses' defences, which prevented them from acknowledging that the things they have to do are so awful that emotional care is required. However, the fact that the nurse cannot be held responsible for the child requiring treatment does not mean she is not, at least in part, responsible for determining how the child manages it. A difference could even be made if the nurses could understand that continuity is an ideal to *aim* for, rather than something we should strive to prevent, and that this should be part of our principles of care. My observations demonstrated that unexpected intrusion from an unfamiliar nurse provoked the greatest anxiety for all parties. Difficulties were evident in trying to help children to manage treatment when scant information of their previous experiences and preparation was available. For staff delivering such potentially damaging treatment, should there not be a proviso of preparation and control—an emotional charter?

Hopkins (1986) described doubting whether it really was of benefit for the child to "face the stark reality" of how painful medical treatment can be. I, at times, felt the same applies to the staff, for whom losing conscious awareness of the awfulness is perhaps a necessary defence. I believe that the need for acknowledgment of the traumatic nature of our work and for some sort of "holding" for the staff has been supported by this study. Copley and Forryan (1997, p. 167) state that the "needs of staff who are the recipients of many felt-to-be unbearable feelings in the service of a containing approach also have to be considered." A regular support or discussion group, where painful truths and awareness could be acknowledged, would be imperative if a more receptive environment were to emerge, helping to safeguard the future psychological well-being of all the many persons involved in this world of children's cancer.

Despite the difficulties, I am optimistic that observational studies can influence nursing practice. Hopefully, in the not too distant future each children's ward will practise individualized patient care and have a written "standard of psychological care" to address these issues.

A standard of psychological care—a proposal

- The families' privacy will be honoured.
- The child will have at least one "named nurse" for the duration of their treatment.
- There will be a one-to-one hand-over between nurses, and an individual nurse will be responsible for each child's care per shift.
- The child will be prepared before any procedure.
- The child will always be informed when a procedure needs to be done, and whenever possible the child will be given some choices during the procedure.
- The parent is not expected, nor encouraged, to physically restrain the child.

- A record will be kept in the child's nursing notes of how they manage procedures.
- Play specialists will be involved with a procedure whenever possible.
- Continuity in nursing care will be the aim.
- Minimum numbers of staff will be involved with the child on a daily basis.
- Both parents and staff will have access to support groups, where time and space is given to think about difficult issues.

C Developing a containing relationship with a child living in a residential setting

Gary Yexley

For the past six years I have worked in a small residential home for ten children between the ages of 5 and 11. My arrival at the home coincided with the start of my Tavistock course, which, I hoped, would contribute to and complement my personal, emotional, and professional development. My role and responsibilities during that time developed to include providing a "keyworking" relationship to one child in particular, whom I will call Tom.

The home was founded by a couple who directed the care and education during most of Tom's stay there. However, a few months prior to Tom's departure, the couple retired, and a new organization took over management of the home. This resulted in a change in emphasis and direction towards a therapeutic community model working psychodynamically, based largely on the work of B. Docker Drysdale and D. W. Winnicott.

Tom

Tom's mother had been 19 years of age at the time of his birth and had a history of psychiatric illness. After a few weeks Tom's mother admitted herself to a psychiatric hospital. Tom and his mother stayed there together for a few days before being transferred to a general ward.

This was to enable Tom's care to be maintained in a more appropriate setting. Tom's mother was diagnosed with postnatal depression, and, as a result, Tom's father provided support by looking after him at the weekends.

When Tom was 7 weeks old, he was placed in foster care, with the intention of returning him home to his mother upon her recovery. This did not happen, as after her release from hospital, Tom's parents became engaged in a cycle of alcohol abuse, domestic violence, and even suicide attempts. Tom was kept in the foster placement before eventually returning home at the age of 6 months.

Tom was then reported to be happy, contented, and responding well to his mother, and for the next two-and-a-half years there was no involvement on the part of Social Services. However, a health visitor continued to monitor Tom's progress and well-being. He was 3 years and 3 months old when his brother was born. It is not clear whether resulting difficulties for Tom were due to an inability of his parents to cope with two children or whether something more deliberately abusive took place. At this time, Tom started going to nursery, but he had difficulties playing with other children. These difficulties increased, with Tom resorting to physical aggression as a way of dealing with his peer relationships. Tom's parents both made suicide attempts, and eventually mother did kill herself. Tom was again placed with foster carers but continued to display challenging and difficult behaviour. Consequently, he moved between various foster carers until he was returned to live with his father prior to starting primary school. Once at school, Tom displayed a combination of emotional, behavioural, and social difficulties and as a result was permanently excluded.

Further disruptions in Tom's life led to the courts finally placing Tom and his brother in the care of Social Services. Tom was now 5½ years old, and for the next two years they moved through multiple foster agency placements, each breaking down. Tom was then, at the age of 7½, separated from his brother and moved to the residential children's home where I work.

Developing a containing relationship with Tom

Upon first meeting Tom, I found it difficult to believe that that he was a child capable of causing such disruption as to warrant a life growing up outside a family—a life living in an institution, looked after by multiple carers, of whom I was now one. I found myself feeling somewhat uncomfortable after having read the background reports on Tom—reports that represented a somewhat stereotypical picture of a child "in care", having as its focus the child as being the "one with the problem", rather than acknowledging all the factors that had contributed to the child's present circumstances. There also appeared to be little understanding of Tom's behaviour. It was represented only as violent and out of control and in no way as a possible communication of disturbed and uncontained feelings or as a reflection of past abusive experiences. It was clear that Tom's situation had presented everyone with complex difficulties. Professionals conveyed their frustration at not being able to identify an environment in which his needs could be met.

I became aware that I was now part of an organization considered to be a positive intervention for him. I was unsure how I was going to fit into a team attempting to understand Tom's difficulties and provide him with containment. I remember feeling troubled by my relative lack of experience and wondered whether I would have felt more confident if I had had children of my own. My work environment also felt somewhat overwhelming to me, with its intense relationships, preoccupations, and attention to detail. The culture and organizational structure of the home was centred largely on the leadership of the founding director. This enabled a consistent level of care to be given to the children and maintained a focus on the primary tasks of care and education.

I was somewhat unprepared for some of the other aspects of working in such an environment while also attending a course that looked at relationships. First, there was the task of understanding the intense projections that I was subjected to in my work with Tom. Second, there were the feelings of envy and rivalry expressed directly and indirectly by colleagues with regard both to my relationship with Tom and to my attendance on the course. I was unsure how I would manage all these feelings and provide a therapeutic benefit to Tom alongside my own personal and professional development.

Fragile beginnings

Despite my early anxieties, I remember being surprised at how much I personally liked Tom. I immediately connected with his interests and found his questions about subjects, including science, interesting and engaging. Tom and I liked playing outside in the garden together or indoors on his favourite computer game. We seemed to be enjoying the beginning of our relationship.

As the days turned into weeks, I began to find it difficult to understand some of Tom's feelings or to gauge his levels of anxiety. Shortly after becoming Tom's keyworker, I noticed, however, that he appeared to react to some situations in an angry and aggressive manner.

> Tom and I were preparing to go to school. We made our way towards the car, and as we approached, I asked Tom to take a seat in the back, and I sat next to him. Tom immediately became angry with me, saying, "Why do you have to sit next to me, don't you trust me?" He continued, "I don't normally have someone sitting next to me!" I replied somewhat defensively that I had wanted to sit next to Tom as I had not seen him much since returning from holiday, but that if he would rather, I could sit somewhere else. Tom did not answer but instead continued to protest, saying that he would "Rather walk than sit next to me!"

I was surprised by how much my presence and possibly also my absence on holiday had affected Tom. I was unprepared for his reaction towards me as well as for my own feelings of anger at this display of rejection. On reflection, I realized that both Tom and I were reacting to my absence, he by distancing himself from a too close relationship and I by feeling I had to keep him close to me. I felt a sense of frustration and guilt as I struggled to understand all this. I wondered, however, if, like me, Tom had been surprised by his response, and whether he was aware of the important communication contained within this interaction about our relationship.

I decided that thinking about Tom's early relationship with his mother might provide me with a valuable insight into what seemed a persecutory and at times even paranoid response from Tom to some situations. I was aware from Tom's file that his mother had suffered from mental health difficulties prior to and after his birth. I began to wonder how this experience might have impacted on Tom as an infant and young child and have affected his ability to develop relationships. I wondered in particular about Tom's mother's capacity to meet his emotional needs, attending to his earliest fears and anxieties. Bion (1967a) suggests that normal development is dependent on a mother's capacity to accept, transform, and make tolerable to the infant primitive feelings, such as that it is dying. But if "the projection is not accepted by the mother the infant feels that its feeling that it is dying is stripped of such meaning as it has. It therefore reintrojects, not a fear of dying made tolerable, but a nameless dread" (p. 116).

With this in mind, I began to wonder whether Tom's early relationship with his mother had provided him with an opportunity to project his early experiences of distress, or whether the pre-occupation with her own emotional difficulties had resulted in an experience for Tom of a mind unavailable to projections. I wondered how this might have influenced Tom's perception of himself. It appeared, however, that I had become someone into whom Tom felt able to project distress. Colleagues and the seminar group helped me to begin to understand that if I was to build a therapeutic relationship with Tom, I would first need to bear the weight of these powerful projections. In doing so, I could provide Tom with an experience of a mind that might perhaps allow him to overcome the consequences of his early deprivation and disappointment.

As my work with Tom continued, our relationship became more intense, and Tom was often angry and aggressive. I also noticed that some of my experiences with Tom appeared similar to the relationship described between him and his father, except that in our interactions the roles were reversed, as I was often placed in the role of the child, with Tom assuming the role of a "bossy father".

Blood, sweat, and tears

Despite these challenges, Tom and I persevered, and after six months there was a shift in our relationship. This was symbolized in a conversation that took place between us following an incident Tom had with a peer over the choice of a video to be watched before settling to bed.

> I went upstairs and could not hear a sound coming from Tom's room; I knocked on the door and entered. Tom was standing just inside the door, and I noticed that he had tears in his eyes. I crouched down to below his eye level and asked him what the matter was.
>
> Tom looked at me, his fists clenched, his body stiff, as though he was about to burst, and said, "You know!" I felt a sense of uselessness, as I didn't know at all. I asked Tom what it was that I was supposed to know, and he reacted to this by becoming even tenser. I said that I did not know how to help him unless he could help me to understand what it was that I was supposed to know. Tom looked directly at me and said, "Things die! Mothers die!"

> At this point I felt a wave of sadness come over me. My eyes filled with tears as I realized what Tom was telling me. He was referring to the video chosen by his peer in which a mother dinosaur dies, leaving her baby dinosaur orphaned. I struggled with the enormity of what Tom had just said to me. I looked at Tom, who appeared to have relaxed his body slightly, and I had the sense that Tom was all too aware of my struggle to find words with which to respond.

This experience marked a major development. It was the first time that Tom had been able to communicate such a deep feeling to me and to involve me in an aspect of his life that was profoundly personal and painful to him. Tom's relationship with me had now developed to accommodate this level of trust.

Although pleased to realize this, I also felt overwhelmed by the intensity of the feelings evoked. My tearful eyes and struggle to find any words left me reflecting on feelings of despair, helplessness, and impotence. I felt that my own development was still in its infancy, although I took some comfort in my ability to help Tom to think about his mother's death. But I also became aware of powerful feelings towards my colleagues and, in particular, the director of the home, feeling angry and frustrated at what I felt were restrictions and expectations imposed on my relationship with Tom as a consequence of the definition of my task. To my mind, these appeared to raise questions about the degree to which my relationship with Tom was supported within the home. I began to think that a culture of dependency on the leader held sway within the home, and I felt uncomfortable at the impact that this had on me. Indeed, I became convinced that I was dealing with a basic assumption group (Bion, 1961) in my work setting.

Bion described basic assumption dependency as an organizational dynamic in which the

> group behaves as if its primary task is solely for the satisfaction of the needs and wishes of its members. The leader is expected to look after, protect and sustain the members of the group, to make them feel good, and not to face them with the group's real purpose. The leader serves as a focus for a pathological form of dependency which inhibits growth and development . . . [Bion, 1961]

However, in discussion with my seminar group, I was able to think about these organizational dynamics and eventually recognize that some of my feelings matched the previous experiences of other professionals involved in Tom's care, in particular the taking up of a protective role towards him and anger with the "neglectful organization". This insight helped me to understand how these feelings could be partly a projection of Tom's own feelings of despair, helplessness, and impotence. I began to realize that I needed to understand more about the professional task with which I had been entrusted and to integrate somehow my experiences of working with Tom with the ideas received from colleagues, the seminar group, and the course.

I realized that it was important to focus on my capacity to think clearly—in other words, maintaining a steadiness of my own in the midst of powerful and intense projections coming from Tom. This appeared to be the vital function with which I could contribute to Tom's development, as well as my own. I felt that it was important for me to be prepared for a close relationship with Tom, without re-enacting the themes of rejection and physical abuse that were features of his early relationships. Bion (1962a) insisted that a certain degree of projective identification is necessary if a child is to communicate with its mother using her as the "container" for the feelings he is unable to bear. The mother responds to the child after unconsciously processing the unbearable feelings. Bion maintained that such processing is the primary way that a mother gets to know her baby.

This understanding prompted me to think more carefully about my responses to Tom and allowed me to find ways in which to begin to talk to him about his difficult and sometimes unbearable feelings. This was illustrated during this interaction.

> Tom and I continued to remove the more delicately placed blocks in turn, aware that the stack could topple over at any time. Tom then bent down to test a block and said, "If I take this one out, the stack will fall down." I agreed and, after thinking for a moment, said to Tom, "You could take that one out, but you would be doing it knowing that the stack would fall down." I followed this statement with the question, "Is that what you would want to happen?" Tom looked up, making eye contact with me, and said, "I could." I responded by repeating his words back to him, saying, "Yes, you could!" Tom looked at the stack and then back to me and said, "But I won't."

I wondered whether Tom felt that knowing him or being with him was somehow dangerous to others. I felt rather unprepared for Tom's testing out my capacity to withstand and, if possible, understand some of his more sadistic projections. His sadistic and revengeful feelings intensified following the loss of an important male figure in his life at the home. This next example illustrates my efforts to understand his feelings of loss at this time, as we went for a walk one day.

> We continued the walk through the wood, and I decided to raise with Tom the possibility of not finding a replacement stick on this trip. I spoke to him, saying, "I suppose it might be possible, Tom, that you might not find another stick on our walk today." Tom did not reply, and I wondered if this notion was too impossible for him to contemplate. I followed my statement by saying; "Well, if we can't find a stick today, then perhaps we might find one on our next walk in the woods." Tom once again did not reply; instead, he drew my attention to a nearby tree, saying, "This one will be OK!" I walked towards Tom and asked him to explain what he meant. Tom explained that he had found a branch on a tree that was suitable. He asked me to break off the branch and attempt to fashion it into a new stick. I decided to follow Tom's request, proceeding to remove the branch from the tree, strip the bark of all loose twigs, and so on. As I finished, I gave the stick to Tom, saying, "There you are, Tom, is that OK?" Tom looked at the stick briefly before beginning to wave it about in a swishing motion. Tom then approached some nearby weeds and nettles and began hitting them with the stick. I waited in anticipation for Tom's appraisal of the new stick, wondering to myself if it would come up to his expectations. I did not have to wait long, as Tom said, "Yeah, this will do for today." I felt an enormous sense of relief and immediately felt more relaxed. Tom continued to hit the weeds and nettles with his new stick for the next ten minutes of the walk. At the end of this time, Tom appeared to lose interest in the stick, handing it to me, saying, "I don't like this stick any more, it's too bendy."

This episode describes a degree of rejection from Tom, possibly due to the rejection felt by him at the loss of an important member of staff. I wondered whether this loss had stirred up feelings of rejection from his past, possibly prompting him to reject aspects of my relationship with him.

Change and transitions

These difficulties within our relationship increased as both Tom and I faced a number of forthcoming changes. These included the home moving to new premises in preparation for the retirement of the director, and the simultaneous changeover to a new management. In addition, there were changes specifically for Tom and myself: Tom was due to have his own planned departure from the home, and I took up a new role within the senior staff team.

I reflected on my many feelings, including those of guilt, as I recognized the impact on Tom of all these changes. I wondered how he must feel, having invested in his relationship with me, only for it to be subjected to a kind of rejection. Despite this, I was encouraged by the way in which Tom continued to initiate ways in which to communicate some of his feelings.

> Tom looked at the cup of water that I was holding and took it from me. He walked into the bathroom and, upon reaching the toilet, tipped the contents of the cup slowly into it. Tom then noticed that the water level in the toilet had not changed. He then made his way to the basket on the bathroom floor that contained a selection of bath toys. He picked up a large plastic bottle and proceeded to fill it up with water from the tap, telling me as he did so that it didn't matter how much water you poured into a toilet, the water level did not go up. Tom walked towards the toilet and tipped the contents of the container in. I watched Tom and felt as though I was being slowly tortured. In addition, I felt hugely saddened. I spoke to Tom and said, "So what you're saying is, that no matter how much water you pour into the toilet, it won't fill up." Tom responded, "Yes" and put the plastic bottle down and left the bathroom.

As I spoke to Tom, I felt as though he understood some of the implication behind my comment. I felt that Tom's response communicated something about the rejection and sadness that he felt at the time of impending transitions and endings. I also felt that however painful his feelings, I had witnessed symbolic play, and an ability to observe the water level closely and formulate a hypothesis.

Tom continued to feel rejected by the staff at the home, including me, and despite my best efforts to maintain a high level of attentiveness, his behaviour and levels of emotional integration deteriorated, and he found it difficult to invest in new staff and peer group relationships. I wondered if he felt that making relationships was almost a kind of torture for him. Tom left the home as planned, and for some time afterwards I felt a combination of frustration, anger, and guilt at the manner in which we had parted. I found it difficult to recognize the positive elements of my relationship with him but, with hindsight, wondered whether Tom was more aware of it in his last communication regarding the containers of water. I concluded ultimately that I had probably played a part in providing him with a "good-enough" experience of a safe, containing adult. I had also needed to recognize and monitor my own limitations and levels of omnipotence in attempting to assess my contribution to Tom's emotional development.

Conclusion

In this chapter, I have focused on the relationship between myself and Tom. This work was carried out over a period of two years and took place within a residential setting. My main theme is the growth of emotional containment, explored through the use of observational material and analysed in relation to the ideas of Klein, Bion, and Winnicott. My understanding of containment developed with the help of colleagues, the seminar group, and the course. This enabled me to focus on the professional task of recreating an experience for Tom of the basic dependence of early relationships, without re-enacting the traumatic elements—including physical abuse—associated with them. I had to struggle to tolerate and understand Tom's most powerful projections, including feelings of anger, sadness at the loss of his mother, guilt, and a desire for revenge for the multiple rejections he had faced during his life. I was sometimes able to reflect back to Tom some of my thoughts about his intense feelings. I have also highlighted the impact of organizational dynamics in my work with Tom, especially my thoughts about the basic assumptions held by the staff group who lived out a dependency culture as a result of the home being run by its founding director. These dynamics revealed the burden of expectation and the dilemmas facing the organization attempting to meet Tom's emotional needs following a life of many painful losses. I have described how my understanding of these dynamics developed, in particular how my feelings resembled those of previous professionals involved in Tom's care, and how they could also be thought about in terms of a projection of Tom's own feelings of despair, helplessness and impotence.

In conclusion, I would like to mention my own self-development. Initially, I found it difficult to understand Tom's communications, which so often took the form of angry and aggressive projections. However, as my work with Tom developed, it provided me with a great opportunity to consolidate my learning of theoretical ideas through their application in very real situations. I was initially unprepared for the powerful nature of the projections to which I was subjected, finding it difficult at times to contain my own feelings. Despite this, I came to regard the experience of working with Tom, colleagues, and the seminar group as both valuable and significant, and as having contributed to my overall emotional and professional development.

CHAPTER SEVEN

Work with vulnerable families

A Working within a refugee community

Fadumo Osman Ahmed

In this chapter I describe the work I do in a community centre, responding to the needs of refugees. Unusually, both staff and clients originate from the same country, most having come to this country within the past 10–12 years. For many, adapting to new circumstances has led to many emotional and exposing moments. It is a community that has experienced loss in a profound way: most of the clients are "single" mothers struggling to bring up 5 or 6 children on their own. It is a life made worse by not knowing what has happened to their husbands, homes, financial assets, and even other children who had become separated in the panicky flight from danger.[1]

There was a paradox in the way the community as a whole dealt with these shocking events: they produced traumatic reactions, but it was difficult for them to be fully acknowledged. I will describe my own attempts to understand quite complex feelings. I became aware that both staff and clients disregarded mental illness, and in fact it seemed to me that the staff deprived their clients of the mental health services they needed, perhaps because it was too painful to face up to these issues.

The institution

There is a small staff that manages to provide an online worker, an outreach worker, and three interpreters. Professional contacts are very widespread, including the Home Office, social security offices, housing department, the local authority, and so forth. Our main aim is to assist families and children to settle in their new country, and, given that clients speak a minimal amount of English, this is a difficult task. There is another complication, in as much as the families have also experienced deep personal and family loss, which in many cases leaves profound emotional turmoil. However, it was difficult for such loss—and, particularly, its emotional consequences—to be acknowledged.

Back at home mental illness was seen as a misfortune and an embarrassment (Bhui et al., 2006). Perhaps for this reason, the organization and its clients did not want to talk about mental illness and its consequences, perhaps for fear of opening what was sitting inside, fear that it might lead to hospitalization and separation from the rest of their family, fear of losing their culture and the shame and stigma that come with it. By contrast, in the United Kingdom there is a greater acceptance of mental illness, and people are more willing to seek help. It seems that the staff of this organization were able to conceal their personal pain and distress by working with and solving the problems of their own community members, and possibly the clients covered up their emotional distress by caring for the family and dealing with immediate services that were needed while settling.

My position was as an outreach worker, which entailed paying home visits, assessing and advising clients who could not come to the centre, such as parents with small children, the mentally ill, and the elderly. During interviews I found myself having, above all, to listen to their problems, rather than to offer advice. I felt that the clients' minds and thoughts were full of pain mixed with fears, and they were therefore not free to take anything in. I wasn't trained to provide counselling or a therapeutic service, but I realized that advice and guidance wasn't enough, as these clients had encountered an enormous trauma and were frightened, isolated, and in mourning.

When with them, I found it difficult to contain my own emotions and protect myself against the impact of their terrible experiences (Whittaker, Hardy, Lewis, & Buchan, 2005). It was perhaps my own difficulty in expressing what I was feeling that helped to put me in touch emotionally with the children of clients. For the most part they suffered in silence, without the opportunity to vent their pain: usually we dealt directly with parents, active on their behalf, and it was this kind of work that could lead to permission being given to act on behalf of children. Here I describe work undertaken with two families following separate crises. Thanks to my having previously established a relationship of some trust, the parents were not afraid to deal with their own and their children's internal and external realities. They were able to manage the painful experiences that accompany such processes as dealing with social services over a long and involved period. This marked a departure from the usual practice of attempting a solution only with the help of elderly members of their community.

Meira

I was contacted by a member of the community who informed me that her neighbour (Lawina) was very concerned that her child Meira (3 years) had been abused by a worker at the local nursery. The following is an account of the telephone conversation:

> Lawina told me that when the children had come home from school and she had come home from shopping, her younger children raced to get their sweets and chocolates, except Meira. Lawina then had asked Meira what had happened to her. Meira didn't respond. Lawina said that she had asked Meira how school was. Meira replied, "I don't like my teacher." Lawina said that she told Meira that she was coming to talk to her when she finished cooking. Lawina said that she felt uneasy while cooking, as the other children played, and Meira was still sitting in the living room. Lawina said that she took Meira into her room and asked why she didn't like her teacher. Lawina then said that Meira had cried and said that her teacher had put a finger in her. Lawina said that she was shocked and couldn't believe the statement. Lawina said that she hugged Meira and while hugging she asked if she could show where. Lawina said that Meira had pointed down. Lawina sounded anxious, and sometimes I couldn't hear what she was saying.

My first decision was that this matter ought not be confined to the local community. I explained that I would phone a colleague paediatrician. There was much anxiety about confidentiality, and I shared this while arranging a visit to the paediatrician.

The first meeting

> Lawina reported that Meira had been examined and that there was no physical damage, and social services were informed to investigate the case. Lawina reported that she had not sent Meira and her younger siblings to school for the past few days. Lawina looked tired and pale, was angry as the school didn't contact her, and was disappointed by the head teacher, whom she described as previously helpful and understanding. Lawina said that a social worker telephoned twice with no interpreter, but Lawina's older son had assisted her. Lawina continued and said that her son was upset and concerned about the situation, as he is close to his brothers and sisters. Another dilemma was that the other three children kept on asking when they were going back to school. Lawina said, "Do you know, today is the third day, and they have not even telephoned." Lawina looked at me straight in the eyes. I felt that she was examining my expressions and body language for a response or reaction.

I explained that when something like that happens, the school and social services have the responsibility to investigate the matter, follow child protection procedures, and then contact families. I added that I felt waiting for a response for three days was too long. However, this issue was very sensitive, and we could not approach the school directly, but with her consent I could contact the Refugee Education Co-ordinator to assist us in this matter. The coordinator's response was that the school and social services were in the process of following child protection procedures, and an interview date was going to be set for Lawina. The coordinator reported that the accused teacher had been a teacher for 16 years. Furthermore, there was no proof that the incident had taken place, only an allegation against a respected teacher.

I felt that communication had broken down and suspected that the chance to develop a healthy relationship between social services and the mother was precarious. The school and social worker appeared to be neglecting Meira's feelings and concentrating on defending the teacher and the school's reputation. It seemed that they did not understand the mother's anxiety and that she was seeking protection for her daughter. I felt the decision not to include Meira and interview her was perhaps because the school and social worker were afraid to reflect on and deal with their own painful emotions.

I also felt that Lawina's description of feeling disappointed with the head teacher perhaps reflected that she was angry and disappointed with Meira, as she had put the family into conflict with the school. There were also family difficulties, since Meira's siblings were angry with her for not being able to go to school.

As a consequence, Lawina acted as if she was able to draw up her own rules and had withdrawn the children from school. When Lawina seemed to be checking on my expression, I felt that she was perhaps trying to find out if I was part of the school and social services and which side I was on.

A week later

> I received a phone call from the social worker, who told me that she understood that I wanted to speak with her about the date of the meeting, but she understood clearly from Lawina that she didn't want any involvement from the community. I explained to the social worker that I was involved with the case from the beginning and that I wasn't coming to compromise the situation but wanted a solution. The social worker was also unwilling to alter the meeting day, which was unsuitable for me.

I telephoned Lawina to explain the telephone conversation that I had had with the social worker. Lawina then said in an angry voice, "That's what happens when a child interprets for you" and told me that her message was that she did not want an interpreter on the day of the meeting, as she was coming with a relative. I advised her that the meeting could take place without me as long as the school provided a support worker and told her to write down the questions that she wanted to ask, and gave her an appointment to come and see us again if she needed to. I struggled to manage my feelings about being excluded.

The feedback from Lawina about the meeting with the school and social services was that she was disappointed with the outcome. The school thought that there was no evidence so far to prove the allegations, and therefore social services had closed the case. Lawina felt that the meeting was a formality and that they had already drawn their conclusions. I felt that the social worker was biased, as she did not give time to build a relationship with the family and had not given adequate time to explore the issue.

Three days later

Social services invited me to assist them and intervene because Lawina wasn't sending the children to school. This suggested to me that her worries, pain, and anger weren't contained. It felt that she could not be in control of the school situation but could control her children.

Reflections

The unfortunate outcome to this case was, in fact, very informative for me. Although there were a number of difficulties, such as the personal pressure on me to belong to "one side" or the other, the incident emphasized the need for the community to have appropriate access to public services, and for a more formal arrangement with statutory services to be developed as a priority so that misunderstandings and prejudices could be overcome.

Faisar

Faisar was 3 at the time of his referral by his mother, Hibak. She said she was experiencing great difficulties, coping with two children under 5, especially as one of them (Faisar) was "handicapped". Unlike the first situation described above, they were in frequent communication with a range of professionals but were feeling quite overwhelmed and confused by the detailed advice given. The felt they needed the support of and intervention by the community.

At a meeting, Hibak told me that Faisar's progress had been normal before he had his MMR immunization at the age of 14 months. He would get up during the night and cry, and because of these disruptions he now slept in his parents' bed. Santhia sleeps with her older sister, and the father sleeps in the living room. In addition, Hibak told me that the health visitor had arranged a nursery for Faisar. However, Hibak said that it was tiring to take Faisar to the nursery for only two and a half hours a day. I felt that Hibak was exhausted and without help. She talked about her feelings of anger around the losses in her life and her distress; she sounded overwhelmed.

> I arranged to pay a home visit. Father, mother, Faisar, and his little sister Santhia were present. The mother, Faisar, and his little sister were in the living room. This meeting happened two weeks after the initial meeting, and during that period I managed to meet with

a local nursery manager who told me that there were vacancies at their nursery and they could think about taking Faisar. Both parents were excited about the news, and I asked if they also wanted support of a social worker and respite care or maybe to first wait to see how we progressed with the nursery. Mother was enthusiastic, but father was unsure. Then mother told me that the appointment for Faisar's Care Planning Meeting had been postponed.

Faisar was sitting on a bicycle very close to the television, watching and giving it all his attention. After a few seconds sitting still on his bike, he looked at the window, and then rode the bike from one end of the room to the other. My first impression was that there was no problem with Faisar's powers of attention, although he was making a wailing noise while he played on his bicycle. Santhia took a scarf from the floor. The father came out of the kitchen and gave a piece of peeled apple to Faisar. Faisar took it with a distracted look and ate it. His father commented, "He doesn't communicate." His father sat on the same sofa as the mother, but also close to Faisar and the television.

While watching the children's programme, Faisar murmured and rocked himself. It seemed that he might have been singing. In addition, Faisar continuously rolled his t-shirt up to his chest and down again. Subsequently, his mother called his name a few times, but he did not look at her. He seemed not to hear his mother at all and appeared distant, with an absent expression. The father then commented in a disappointed way that nine months earlier Faisar had waved and said "bye-bye" to him, and on the same day he said, "Give me", and this had continued for three days. He had then stopped talking again. Faisar wasn't looking at us, but I was wondering how much of the conversation he was taking in and the effect or the impact of it. I was also thinking of the frustration and the anger he probably felt inside as he was not able to express his feelings.

Afterwards his little sister played with her parents. She stood on the sofa that they were sitting on. She then went behind them, touched their heads alternately, and pulled her mother's headscarf from her head and tried to put it on hers. The father tickled her, and the group laughed. Faisar stopped playing and stared at them with what seemed to me to be a profoundly sad look. He had not participated in the game but kept on looking at them, but neither of his parents asked him to join in. Regardless of his busy surroundings, Faisar seemed lonely. I felt that there was no warmth and understanding from his parents that could include him. Nobody seemed to think about him, and I wondered whether his parents were thinking that he was as good as dead to them because of the MMR and were therefore unable to hold him in mind. I felt very affected by the despair of the parents, but I felt I needed to bear it without rejection. I felt that I held on to the possibility of communication. I had observed that there was a box full of toys right next to Faisar, but he never made an effort to get any out. Sitting on his bike, he stared at or through the window, and I wondered if it was too painful to stay tuned into this setting and that therefore he was in search of a quiet place, or if he was experiencing a state of more profound withdrawal. I wondered whether the withdrawal was linked in some way to the presence of his younger, competent sister.

Finally, Faisar rode his bike again from one of the room to another, hardly making eye contact with any of us. Again I was interested. I wondered at the seeming absence of curiosity, the wish to explore. Was he having a "bad day", or was it something more permanent? I felt like going near him, talking to him, and diverting him from his lonely existence before I left, but Faisar went to the window and moved a toy from one end to the other. I said, "Bye-bye, Faisar", but he did not turn.

Linking notes

A few weeks later Faisar had his Multidisciplinary Assessment Report meeting. Present were Faisar's paediatrician, a health visitor, a physiotherapist, the father, the mother, and myself. My role was to support the parents and facilitate communication. I had not met any of the professionals before, but I had read their reports, and the parents had talked about them. Faisar and his little sister were left with a neighbour.

During the meeting, it was said that Faisar had a severe delay in speech and had not much social interaction. The paediatrician said that when examining Faisar, he had become upset, and he himself had thus been unable to complete tasks such as measuring his head. However, he had found that Faisar's gross neurological condition was normal. It was noted that Faisar had some communication skills and that there were no concerns about his gross motor skills. The health visitor said that when she had visited the family in their house, Faisar had recognized her, and he was calm during her visit. It was also reported that once in the clinic he had picked up a pair of scissors and had tried to cut his hair. His mother then informed the meeting that he had had a haircut the previous day! The team emphasized that there were possible autistic spectrum features and suggested that he could benefit by doing routine tasks. The physiotherapist and the health visitor were assigned to assist Faisar and do routine tasks with him. I reported that I had succeeded in arranging a nursery place for Faisar. However, his mother said he would find it too tiring to be in a nursery for two and a half hours every day, given his behaviour.

Second home visit

Mother, Faisar, little sister Santhia, and the older brother (10) were present. Father was not there. When I went into the living room, Faisar was standing on the sofa. He touched the window, got off the sofa, and ran out of the room. He went into the bathroom, touched the sink, and came back to the sofa. He ran back and forth, making an "eeeii, eeeiii" noise. He seemed to enjoy climbing up and down. I greeted mother and Santhia. I then went near Faisar and greeted him, but he did not look at me or give any signs of being aware of my presence. He continued running. The mother was sitting on an armchair with Santhia on her lap, and there were toys scattered on the floor.

Faisar looked very thin. I had not seen him for nearly three weeks, but I could see the change in his weight. I recalled the health visitor's comment that he could remember when things were repeated. So I changed seats in order to interact with Faisar, and I sat on the sofa where he kept running from, in the hope of engaging with him. Once I thought Faisar would step on the toys on the floor and hurt himself because he seemed not to be paying attention to what was on the floor. I shook a cylindrical toy with beads inside and offered it to him. He looked at me with a tense expression, perhaps wondering who I was. I asked if he wanted to play, and although he did not join in, he looked less tense. I called his name and went in front of him, holding a different toy this time—a spade and a bucket. I then took a car with flashing lights and wheeled it on the floor. Faisar sat on the floor, and with an interested look he held the car. I told him the colours of the car—red and yellow—and while he was staring at it, my fear was that he would never engage with me. I wondered if he recognized me as having been part of the group in the previous meeting, as I was in the same room with him and sat not far from his Mum and father.

After a few minutes Faisar went to his Mum and sat on her lap. Facing her, he held her neck tight. His mother repeated, "Gently—gently" while trying to take his hands from around her neck. She then kissed him and asked what he wanted. She rocked him, but he was aggressive. He then made a mournful noise. The mother called out for her older daughter and asked her to bring biscuits for him and Santhia. I felt that mother understood his signals but conveyed the wrong message: instead of stopping and showing him how to ask for something, she rocked and kissed. Afterwards she went to the kitchen to prepare food for the children, and while in the kitchen, she asked Faisar and Santhia to play together. Faisar had the biscuits in his right hand, and while eating, he started running back and forth. I tried to stop him and get him to sit down, and asked if he wanted to play with his sister and me, but he made it clear that he did not want to, and I let him go.

The mother brought a sandwich and an apple for Faisar, and soup and bread for Santhia. The mother informed me that Faisar did not like moist food. "His bread or rice has to be dry; he likes meat and doesn't have a problem eating." I then asked if he had grown taller or if he had lost weight? "He has lost a lot of weight, because he is running most of the time", said the mother in a disappointed way. Referring to her husband and older daughter, I then said that she had a lot of help from them, but she said that father had left the family since the last meeting. I was shocked to hear this and wondered whether mother was feeling that Faisar was to be blamed. Following this meeting, there was a period of impasse. Mother wanted Faisar to attend nursery full-time and was concerned about the length of time Faisar spent watching television when at home. She was convinced that his social skills would improve and that he would benefit from a place without television. However, the nursery had advised Faisar's parents that they could not have him full-time because of his lack of communication and his difficulties in integrating with other children. They would have to wait until the education authority provided a one-to-one worker.

An educational psychologist assessed Faisar at the nursery after a further delay, and she suggested that he should continue attending part-time. In the meantime the nursery should help him with some specific tasks until her next visit. Mother was unhappy with this decision and asked me if together we could meet the nursery manager. I had the impression that, because the educational psychologist had visited the nursery when the parents were not around, the mother felt that her son's needs and their requests had not been taken into account. I also sensed that mother felt that the ultimate decision rested with the nursery manager.

Visit to the nursery

The appointment was on a Monday. Faisar was to start nursery at 9.15 am, and therefore I had suggested meeting them at home at 9.00 am. When I went, mother and Faisar were ready. Father, who came to support, stayed at home to look after Santhia. I understood from mother that father comes around to help. Mother had told me that she had found it difficult to settle Faisar the previous week after the half-term holiday because he had missed the first three days of the week before because he had flu, and she feared that on that day, too, he would not stay at nursery. I then told her that I could stay a bit longer with Faisar after we finished the meeting, if the nursery agreed.

> On the way to the nursery, Faisar did not have a problem walking or holding his mother's hand. He had neither a cheerful expression, nor a sad one. He made brief eye contact when his mother took his hand and did not complain. He looked taller and a little relaxed. When near the nursery, mother pointed to a grassy area in front of us and told me, "He likes to climb the little hills", and predicted, "Watch, he will run from us", but Faisar did not.
>
> When we went into the nursery, I was introduced to two members of staff and their two groups of children. Most of the children greeted Faisar, but he did not respond and was clinging on to his mother. We then went into the manager's office. She stood up to greet us. Faisar, without being invited, sat on a chair. The rest of us remained standing. The manager, shrugging her shoulders, said, "We haven't received any reply yet. Have you?" I said, "No." The manager continued, "Clearly it is about funds; the Education Authority wants the Social Services to fund his place, and vice

versa." This was not the first time that this financial issue had come up, and automatically I looked at mother. She frowned, and her bottom lip was tightly between her teeth. Faisar, sitting on the swivel chair, had his hands on the side of the chair, and his posture was upright. I wondered if he was feeling rather grandiose. This time he moved the swivel chair from side to side again and again. The manager then added, "I have another child, older than Faisar, that the Education Authority insisted went to primary school in January, but he was not yet ready and would not get the attention that he needs. Therefore I advised his mother to let him stay until November."

I then asked the manager if she could update us on Faisar's position. I explained that the parents had been confused about all the agencies that appeared not to be linking up. For example, the educational psychologist did not inform the parents when she was visiting Faisar at the nursery. Consequently, after she had assessed him, she had not sent any feedback to the parents, and the little information they had was what the nursery manager had given to them, although the parents were grateful for this. The manager explained that it was myself and the speech and language therapist who had referred Faisar to the unit, and yet he, the manager, was expected to arrange referral to social services and education. The nursery manager continued, "I clearly told the speech and language therapist that it wasn't my responsibility and she had to do it, and now I feel that that is why there is a delay in his getting a full-time place." I felt confused and excluded and not part of the system, because in my previous contacts with the manager she had not told me about this matter.

Faisar was still sitting on the swivel chair; he slowly moved from side to side, and he was touching and feeling the synthetic material on the side supports, occasionally putting his hands on his ears. I asked the manager what her opinion was about Faisar having a full-time place. She said, "Faisar would benefit from a one-to-one worker, and until that happens, we can't have him." I asked if she had mentioned this to the educational psychologist. She said, "Oh, yes! I also wrote a letter." I then asked if she could give us a copy of that letter, as I was going to write a letter to the child development team and to the Education Authority. She then strongly said, "I did send it. I don't have a copy." I felt puzzled

> about this and tried to control my wish to question so as not to pass my anxiety on to the mother. It seemed to me that the manager wanted to keep Faisar part-time even though they could not meet his needs.
>
> The manager then tried to explain to us more about why they could not have him full-time and reported that the day the educational psychologist had visited, they had fewer children. Under the new regulations they could only take two 2-year-olds who needed special attention and to have their nappies changed.
>
> We then went to join Faisar's group, who were doing different activities. Loud greetings came from his teachers and from some of the children. Faisar clung to his mother and did not want to join the group. Mother and I greeted them back, but Faisar held his mother's leg, burying his face in her thighs and refusing to take his jacket off. His mother then said, "I am not going, I will stay with you", but before she finished he was screaming and stamping his feet on the floor. He continued trying to prevent his mother taking his jacket off. He held on to her right leg, clinging on to her as she went to the cloakroom and hung up his jacket.
>
> He continued to cry for some time, holding on to his mother. No nursery staff approached us to help mother or defuse Faisar's anger. After a few minutes, it was teatime. One of the workers came to take Faisar outside, and extending her right arm, she said, "Come, you like playing outside." Then Faisar and his mother went along. I hesitated to join them, as mother did not invite me. Mother then came back after a few minutes and told me, in a commanding tone, "Let's go while he is busy." I almost felt that she wanted to pull my arm, and we left the nursery. At the same time I found her actions disturbing and felt I was colluding with her. I also felt very strongly that while Faisar might well need someone to help him in a practical way on a one-to-one basis, he clearly needed to be in contact with someone who could understand his communications better than I could.

I felt that Faisar would benefit from some specialist help. After a complex process, it was possible to arrange work for the parents and individual work for Faisar. I was left to reflect on a difficult but rewarding time during which I came to understand powerfully the pressures that can be placed on institutions struggling to cope with limited resources. It also became clear that I was perceived by the community and statutory services alike as a discomfiting figure. The community regarded me as someone who knew how to get access to resources but felt that they could not be sure that I would be partisan. Statutory services, on the other hand, could easily make the assumption that I was totally absorbed in the community and lacked objectivity. Negotiating a way through the small space this left me was often painful.

Note

1. The issue of underachievement by pupils of this community is described in more detail by Ali & Jones (2000).

B Providing a play setting for children visiting parents in prison

Margherita Castellani

In this chapter I explore the experience of being a play-worker within the precincts of an inner-city prison. I will reflect on the experience of working within this setting before describing in some detail my work with two children, to whom I will refer as Sophia and Mark. As is mostly the case, they were seen for a short space of time, but, despite the challenging circumstances, they were able to make use of a space for thinking and feeling. Through their play and drawings they were able to get in touch with their feelings and to confront their family's situation.

The setting of the playroom within a prison had a significant impact both on the children themselves and on how I worked. I will describe the situation of the prison by explaining the route a child would take to get the playroom. Through an adult visitor's eyes, the route would not seem particularly daunting, even though it contains necessary security measures for anyone coming in from the outside. But what would a child make of a route that started off in the visitor's centre, where bags are left, continues through electronic doors, glass screens, metal detectors, sometimes dogs for drug inspection, arriving finally in the visiting area—a large rectangular room with a number of tables for families? The playroom is a pleasant, self-contained part of the visitors' room. It is well equipped with toys, books, and art materials, but it may perhaps be difficult for children to take in the appearance of the room while still being caught up in the journey itself.

Before entering the playroom, children need to be registered by their mother or carer. They are then free to go back and forth from the visitors' area to the playroom. The number of children in the playroom varies a great deal, from 1–2 when it is quiet, up to 10–15 during weekends and holidays. There is one play coordinator in charge of the playroom and three to four part-time play-workers. For security reasons the playroom can only be open if there are two play-workers available. If this is not the case, then the one play-worker works in the visitors' room with a box of toys. We see more of the children of remand prisoners, who are allowed daily visits, than those of convicted prisoners, who are restricted to two visits a month.

Play-workers are with the children during visits, which last for approximately one and a half hours, allowing the parents some time alone. We try to provide a more relaxed atmosphere, perhaps achieving an element of normality in an otherwise stressful environment. Over the two years of working in this setting, I have gained a growing awareness of the opportunities, but also the limitations, of my role as a play-worker. I do not have access to the prisoners' files and therefore remain unaware of the period of time during which a child will be visiting the prison. Visits tend to take place on an irregular basis, so that there is little opportunity for continuity in my relationships with the children. In most cases I get to see a child once and then never again. On busy days it is frustrating not to be able to attend to the individual needs of the children. On the other hand, my role as a play-worker enables me to support children during visits, giving them my attention and helping them to express painful and confused emotions.

Visiting children tend to refrain from talking about their experience of having a parent or close relative in jail. They seldom ask questions about officers, gates, and bars, and they hardly ever use the word "prison". This attitude reflects a concern among the families of prisoners about the stigma of incarceration. There is an expectation for children to downplay their painful feelings, avoiding any direct reference to their fathers' imprisonment, a forbidden topic, threatening to throw a bad light upon the family. Parents often do not tell their children the truth about their father's whereabouts: they say that he is staying in a hospital, in a factory, in college, and so on. A 6-year-old once told me that he had a secret he could not tell his mother. He knew that his father was in jail, but he could not tell her, as "she believed that Daddy was in hospital" and she would have been too upset had he told her the truth.

Bowlby observed the difficulties that children have in dealing with experiences that their parents do not wish them to know about. He writes, "the scenes and experiences that tend to become shut off, though often continuing to be extremely influential in affecting thought, feeling and behaviour, [are] those that parents wish their children not to know about" (Bowlby, 1979, p. 101). A main challenge in my role as a play-worker has been to find ways of helping the children to have a more truthful experience while not contradicting or challenging parental explanations.

This state of denial, as a defence against a painful reality, is reflected in the behaviour of the staff. There is a tendency among play-workers to emphasize the "happy" and "nice" aspects of play, avoiding the full impact of disturbing and difficult feelings. I am reminded of Peter Speck writing about "chronic niceness" in relation to staff caring for dying people (1999). He explains how negative and painful feelings get split off and denied while a collective fantasy arises in which "staff are nice people, who are caring for nice dying people, who are going to have a nice death in a nice place" (1999, p. 97). I often sense a similar attitude—an unconscious wish to give an hour of nice play to some nice children, in a nicely decorated playroom. The desire is to leave a distressing, "not-nice" world behind in the visitors' room, keeping the playroom an "uncontaminated" space for "nice" experiences—a protective bubble within a pain-filled institution. Isabel Menzies Lyth talks about a "social defence system" adopted by staff facing high levels of stress. She states that its main characteristic "is its orientation to help the individual avoid the experience of anxiety, guilt, doubts and uncertainty" (1997, p. 63). She remarks that although collective defences can alleviate anxiety, they do not promote growth.

The following episodes, which took place during my first few months at the prison, illustrate my struggle to keep thinking for myself rather than getting drawn into a state of denial.

> There were three children in the playroom. George, a 6-year-old, was standing still in front of the window, staring out through some plastic binoculars. He appeared anxious, in a state that seemed to exclude everything except the grim view outside the window. Robert, a 5-year-old, was wandering around the room aimlessly. Julian, also 5 years old, was sitting on the floor, reading

> a book. There was an oppressive, emotionally flat atmosphere in the room. Mary, the play coordinator, suggested that we all sang a song together. Julian agreed, looking excited. Robert joined in the singing but without any real enthusiasm. George kept staring outside the window, paying no attention to what was going on in the room.

I remember feeling torn between Mary's suggestion to join in the singing, perhaps to escape from the sense of oppression that I was experiencing, and staying with my experience of that oppression, uncomfortable though it might have been. Later, during my work discussion seminar, we reflected upon my role as a play-worker and questioned whether my task was to distract and to cheer up the children, or whether it was to help them to express their real feelings and provide them with an appropriate response. I slowly began to realize that only by keeping in touch with my own feelings could I start helping the children to make sense of their own experience of visiting a jail. The work discussion seminars helped me to keep engaging with my thinking self and to define the different attitudes that Mary and I had towards our work.

Sophia

I met Sophia some ten months after I had started my work at the prison. She was a 6 year old, with long, curly reddish hair, large green eyes, and delicate features—an angelic face. She was shy and extremely cautious in the way she spoke and moved.

> As I was the only play-worker, I could not open up the playroom and could only sit with a box of toys in a corner of the visitors' room. There was one girl sitting at a table with two women and an inmate who was talking extremely loudly. . . . I walked up to their table to tell the girl that there were some toys at the opposite end of the room and that she could join me to play whenever she felt like it. The prisoner replied in a rage, accusing me of trying to take his daughter, whom he had not seen for a long time, away from him. I felt anxious and attacked. I explained to him that it was only a suggestion and that the girl could spend as much time as she wished with her father during the visit. The man replied that if it was just a suggestion, then it was all right and raised his thumb to make an OK sign.

Sophia's father immediately identified me with the institution of the prison and attacked me. My feeling of anxiety about having invaded the family privacy may have been a projection of the father's own sense of being controlled by an intrusive institution. I was perhaps made to feel some of his concerns and trepidation. My acceptance of his negative feelings and reassurance that he could have a choice about how to handle his daughter seemed to help him to feel more in control, less persecuted, and therefore more willing to accept my presence.

> I went back to my table and was joined shortly afterwards by the girl. She sat down next to me, staring silently ahead of her with a distant gaze. . . .
>
> Sophia took some pencils out of the toy box and began making a drawing for her father. In a low voice, very much in contrast with her father shouting, she explained to me what she was drawing: an angel, a blue sky, a large bright sun, and a meadow. Sophia said that she had just begun her summer holiday but that she very much wished that school was still on. There was a sad expression on her face. I told Sophia that at times it is easier to be at school than at home and that probably things were difficult at home. She nodded. . . .

Sophia was able to distance herself from direct contact with her father, at a moment when she may have felt overwhelmed by his angry feelings, leaving her no space. The angel and the sunny blue sky may have indicated a denial of a painful reality, but also the expression of a sense of hope, necessary to persevere. It is interesting to note that after having made this "bright" picture, Sophia was then able to reflect upon her "dark" circumstances at home. Perhaps by holding on to a benevolent object, she could face some painful feelings of loss.

The following passage portrays Sophia's urge to gain understanding about what was happening to her. Melanie Klein used the term "epistemophilic instinct"—the thirst for knowledge—which, she believed, was present from birth. In addition, Klein postulated a "longing for insight", an innate desire to understand one's own internal world (1961).

> . . . Sophia asked me whether I was "Christian or Catholic" and said that she was Christian but did not go to church. She explained to me that she was Irish and that her family were Travellers and

> lived in a trailer. She then added that I looked like a Traveller. I made a comment about Sophia's feeling that we were getting to know one another, perhaps as if we were part of the same family. She continued, saying, "You know, my Dad lives in a crystal palace. It is all shiny and golden inside. I have been with him in the crystal palace, it is a beautiful place." Sophia asked me whether I believed her father lived in a crystal palace, adding that her family had told her so. She said that, if I did not believe her, she was going to ask her Dad. She repeated the same question, and I hesitated, uncertain about what to say. I felt anxious and at a loss for words. Sophia rushed to her father and came back, saying that dad said that he did live in a crystal palace. I told Sophia that she might like to make a drawing of the crystal palace. She agreed with enthusiasm. She drew three tall adjacent towers, a little door on the central one, and some Xs in place of windows. She then added a very large building, which she said was a church. . . .

Sophia's comment about me looking like a Traveller felt like an acknowledgement of contact being established between us. Her insistent questioning about my belief in the crystal palace may have indicated a conflict between her wish for knowledge and a desire to leave things unknown, in order to protect herself or her parents from an unpalatable truth.

I realized that the feelings of anxiety and helplessness evoked in me were a projection of Sophia's own distress and anxieties, which I was able to receive, given that she was unable to think things through at the time. Bion suggests that a stepping stone in an infant's normal development is the experience of a mother—a container—who can receive her child's projected distress into herself—the contained—and hold it, give it meaning and subsequently return it to the infant in a bearable form (Bion, 1959). My task with Sophia was to contain some of her anxieties and doubts, think about them—and later, as we shall see, comment on them.

By making a drawing of the crystal palace, Sophia continued thinking about her experience in the prison. She remarked astutely that the crystal palace was very similar to the entrance gate of the building we were in. I suggested that perhaps people had to stop and pray in the big church she had drawn, before they could leave the crystal palace. She nodded. I thought about that church, wondering whether it was a place of redemption or of judgement. Sophia went on to make more drawings for her father, rushing to bring him the ones she had finished and then returning to my table. In all of them there was an angel. I thought that Sophia might have a reparative mission towards her father, wondering whether she felt responsible for his incarceration. As she was about to finish one of her drawings, Sophia complained about being messy and said that she wanted to be neat—"like you" she added. I remember feeling surprised by how rapidly Sophia had associated me with an idea of "neatness". I told her that she might feel messy because there were so many things she was struggling to understand, like the crystal palace. I commented on how hard it must be having so many questions and no answers. Later on, during the work discussion seminar, we wondered whether Sophia's remark about my being "neat" expressed her feeling that I had not been damaged by her projections or by her father's. I could experience her distress and yet remain intact.

Sophia spent the remaining part of the visit doing a jigsaw puzzle, perhaps in an attempt to create some structure out of a fragmented experience. When the visit was about to end and her mother called her to go and say goodbye to her father, Sophia hesitated, suddenly looking more anxious, then insisted on helping me put all the toys away before returning to her family's table. I told Sophia that it may be hard to be leaving Daddy, adding that perhaps she felt that we had not had enough time together to think about her.

I felt that Sophia had found a safe place for exploring her situation and would have liked more of the attention I had given to her. I found myself struggling with the limitations of my role as a play-worker, wishing I could do more for her. Perhaps I was wanting to become a sort of "saviour" figure too, to "solve" things rather than tolerate a state of uncertainty. Nevertheless I felt I had been able to give Sophia an experience of containment, perhaps helping her to make her journey into the "crystal palace" a less threatening experience.

Mark

I met Mark towards the end of my time as a play-worker. He was 6 years old, very thin, almost waif-like. I was immediately struck by his restless, scrutinizing dark eyes. He stormed into the playroom accompanied by his mother, who asked me if I could "keep Mark", as she needed to talk to her husband. She struck me as an anxious woman who could not cope with Mark and needed help in looking after him.

Mark sat in the wooden car, pretending to be driving. He appeared totally engaged in this activity, over-excited but anxious. He turned the steering-wheel, vigorously leaning his torso from one side of the car seat to the other, making a loud revving sound. I approached Mark and asked him where he was driving to but got no answer, only the same insistent revving sound. After a short while he looked at me and in an excited voice said, "I don't know where I am driving to, I just want to drive." I told Mark that it seemed that he was driving away from the playroom, which perhaps he did not like very much. He went on with the "speed-driving", ignoring me. I asked him whether he was trying to drive away from me? Again, I got no answer, only the revving sound. I felt that Mark had switched off from the reality around him, retreating into a state of isolation as a way of alleviating anxiety. My initial attempts at reaching him were in vain. Through the incessant physical activity, the "speed-driving", Mark seemed to be holding himself together, avoiding the full impact of a painful situation. This first contact with Mark made me feel helpless and rejected. Nevertheless, I realized that perhaps Mark was communicating something to me. He was making me experience what it was like for him to be visiting a jail and to feel frustrated and confused, possibly excluded from his parents' meeting next door or rejected by his imprisoned father. Mary Boston, writing about this mechanism of reversing an unpleasant event, suggests that

> all the children, at times . . . made their therapists feel useless, rejected, abandoned . . . precisely the experiences and feelings which the patients themselves found intolerable or hard to bear. This reversal of painful experience seems very important in trying to understand children who do not find it easy to communicate with words. [Boston, 1983, p. 58]

> Mark got up from the wooden car and wandered around the room for a few minutes, looking at the toys, then stopped by the box containing the plastic monsters. He took one monster out of the box, only to dismiss it, dropping it back into the box. He repeated the same action over and over again, with different monsters. I told Mark that he seemed to like dropping the toys then added that, perhaps, he felt that his mother had dropped him in the playroom. He glanced at me fleetingly, smiling nervously.

I felt that Mark was communicating to me his experience of feeling "dropped" by his parents in a very concrete way. He seemed to be getting some pleasure by turning his passive experience into an active one—he was doing the dropping. Mark's fleeting smile, following my comment about his liking for throwing toys on the floor, gave me a feeling that I had got through to him.

The next sequence portrays in a vivid way some of Mark's preoccupations about visiting the jail.

> He took a posting box from a shelf and spent some time inserting the different plastic shapes, then struggled to get them out. He repeated this action several times, seeming very absorbed in this task. I told Mark that it was easy to put things into the box, harder to take them out. Without looking at me, he uttered to himself "hard". A bit later he grabbed one of the small plastic monsters and put it inside the box, then struggled to take it out. Forcefully shaking the box in the air, he cried out, "It is trapped, it doesn't come out!" I remarked that it might be scary for the monster to be stuck inside the box. He said, "Yes, it is scary." I suggested that perhaps he—Mark—was feeling scared in case he might not be able to get out of the playroom. For a second he froze, then turned away from me. I felt anxious about what I had just said to him.

In this scene Mark shows a capacity to use play material to explore his situation with me. He appears to be confronting the reality of his father as a "monster" trapped in the prison. He may also be expressing his own anxieties about becoming a prisoner himself.

Later I thought about my comment about Mark feeling scared and felt that my words had been premature. He seemed ready to hear that the monster was scared but suddenly looked distressed when I suggested that *he* might also have been scared. I felt that Mark had experienced my comment as threatening and wondered whether I should have simply encouraged him to explore his worried feelings about the monster, without reference to himself.

A week later Mark returned. For the first ten minutes he rushed from one toy to another in a seemingly aimless way.

> He rushed to the box containing the small cars, saying that he wanted to play cars, then moved to the sand tray, starting to play with a bucket and shovel. A minute later he rushed to the home-corner, saying that he wanted to play dolls, then pointed at a large plastic teapot up on a shelf, asking me if I could get it for him. He

> was going so fast that it was impossible for me to follow what he was doing. I told Mark that he didn't seem sure about what he wanted to do.

As he walked into the playroom, once again Mark appeared to be divorced from the things around him. The different toys he took up and then put down seemed to have no meaning for him. Mark's "chaotic" style of play made me feel overwhelmed. Nevertheless, I was aware that Mark was expressing something of his unsettled state of mind, and that my task was to contain his confused feelings, thinking about his restless play, and later comment upon it, rather than encourage him to engage in a specific activity.

Mark wandered restlessly around the room for some time and then said that he wanted to do a painting. He sat at the easel and asked me for some blue and black paint. He painted a skimpy blue "creature", which, he said, was a "budgie", against a black background. He went on to explain to me that he used to have a budgie, but that it had died, adding in a pensive tone, "He was my friend." I was struck by Mark's painting as a poignant depiction of loss and wondered whether he had ever overheard the slang phrase "doing bird". I decided to follow Mark's own pace and to comment upon the death of his budgerigar, rather than introducing the separation from his father. I told him that he must have felt very sad when his "budgie" had died, and that it was hard to separate from a friend. Mark remained silent for some time and finished his painting. Later he asked me how to spell "Dear Daddy, come home soon." He wrote it at the bottom of the painting and rushed to give it to his father. He spent the remaining part of the visit sitting at his parents' table.

Mark thus began to face up to feelings of loss in relation to a distant and safer event—the death of his budgerigar—and later on, as the experience felt less overwhelming, he could start thinking about the separation from his father, expressing his wish for him to return home.

I saw Mark once again a couple of weeks later. He remained in the playroom only for a short time, as he and his mother had to leave the prison earlier than expected: for various reasons, mainly security, visits can come to an abrupt end. It was a painful interaction, which left me filled with a deep sense of grief and sadness.

> He rushed into the playroom and urgently told me that he wanted to do a painting for his father. He sat at the easel and painted

> three very primitive figures, then made a comment, saying "You see, these are the good men." He went on to paint a few more figures, which, he said, were "bad" ones. Suddenly his state of mind seemed different: he looked anxious, on the verge of becoming distressed. He dipped his brush into the black paint and began to block out the figures he had painted. In a rage he tore up his painting and threw it into the bin. I felt anxious, struggling to make sense of Mark's sudden change of mood. I suggested that perhaps he wanted to keep the "bad" and the "good" men separate from one another, and that when they got mixed up together, he felt that they had all turned bad, that the painting had turned bad, and that perhaps he—Mark—had turned bad too. Without looking at me, he said, "Go away." I told Mark that perhaps he felt that I had turned bad too. He got up from his chair and sat in the wooden car, pretending to be driving and making his insistent revving sound.
>
> A few minutes later Mark's mother came into the playroom and told him that they had to leave. He began crying, saying that he didn't want to go, that he wanted to do another painting. . . . Mother replied that they were going to miss their train, grabbed him by an arm, and dragged him away.

That day I left the prison overwhelmed by the feeling that I had not done enough for Mark and his mother. My feeling of helplessness may have been a reflection of their own feelings at the premature curtailment of their visit. In Mark's painting there was an attempt to differentiate the "bad" figures from the "good" ones and to create a sense of order. I felt that Mark was flooded with persecutory feelings as a result of the collapse of this precarious differentiation. Klein's idea of splitting as a primitive defensive mechanism against overwhelming anxieties came to mind. Klein postulated that splitting was clearly linked with persecutory feelings, believing that painful events increase persecutory anxieties. She suggested that

> unpleasant experiences . . . in the young child, especially the lack of happy and close contact with loved people, increase ambivalence, diminish trust and hope and confirm anxieties about inner annihilation and external persecution. [Klein, 1940: 347]

I wondered how the experience of having a father in prison—a father whom society had defined as "bad"—impinged in Mark's inner world on his belief in a good parental object and on his own goodness.

Mark was able to engage in a process of mourning, allowing some distressing feelings to emerge. He could sustain a sober, reflective state of mind, but whenever the anxiety became overwhelming, he retreated into "speed-driving". Sophia, on the other hand, had been desperately colluding with her father's story, employing manic defences against an unbearable reality.

Conclusion

In this chapter I have tried to portray some of the difficulties a child of a prisoner may be facing: confusion over father's incarceration and whereabouts; lack of communication within the family; feelings of guilt and loss; the fear of being turned into a prisoner; and identification with a "bad" father.

I believe that the identification with a "bad" father is a particular risk. We know that children of offenders are far more likely than other children to enter the criminal justice system (Johnston, 1992). There is a desperate need for support for the families of prisoners, providing them with a thinking space for processing their experience. My work was a small contribution to this task.

C Emotional numbing and mindlessness as a phenomenon in residential assessment work

Stuart Hannah

This chapter describes my experience of attending work discussion seminars while I was working as a deputy manager in a local authority family resource centre.

Drawing upon data from presentations in work discussion seminars, I identify themes and developments in my practice and illuminate these with reference to key psychoanalytic ideas and concepts. I endeavour to describe, on reflection, how my work practice benefited from an "added dimension" provided through the experience of work discussion.

I attended these weekly seminars during my pre-clinical child psychotherapy training. I use vignettes from three different pieces of work written up soon after the event for presentation in these seminars, with a view to conveying how my thinking and practice developed as a consequence of this experience. I begin with an example of family assessment work, which I see as illustrating crisis, projections, and containment. I then describe a further piece of family assessment work and link it to the concepts of dysfunction, splitting, and bizarre objects. The final example is an experience within a staff meeting of discussing the needs of one of the adolescents, which I use to discuss role clarification and primary task definition. I conclude with reflections on my greater capacity to track emotionality as a result of the reflective space the work discussion seminars offered me.

Context

Each piece of work described took place in a local authority family resource centre undertaking the dual tasks of comprehensive residential family assessment work alongside short- to medium-term residential assessment work with "looked-after" adolescents. These centres are in-borough resources (owned and managed by social services) whose referrals come from the district social workers. Most referrals are of families about whom there are serious doubts regarding the parents' ongoing capacity to meet their children's needs. The adolescents are usually being "looked after" for the first time following family breakdown, and most require longer-term foster family placements. The assessment task is, therefore, often focused upon assessing their "fosterability".

Crisis, projection, and containment in family assessment work

Four months into my new job as deputy manager and about six months into my attendance at work discussion seminars, I undertook this piece of family assessment work with Carla, the mother of 6-month-old Natalia, and her father, Piero. Carla was diagnosed as suffering from bipolar and personality disorders, and her relationship with Natalia's father had been violent and sexually abusive. The following is part of a write-up made at the time.

> At about 6.25 p.m. Carla walks briskly into the kitchen, with Natalia in her arms. Her hair is wet, as she has just been in the bath. Natalia is wearing a yellow sleepsuit with a small blue teddy emblem on the front. Carla's eyes are wide open as she says to me, rather frantically, "I haven't been to the doctor's yet and it's nearly half past six and Piero's meant to be coming but he isn't anymore. I might as well be a single mother." As she speaks, her eyes begin to well up with tears. "I don't know what to do, he is just leaving us on our own and taking no responsibility." Carla has run out of her lithium medication, and the doctor's surgery is due to close at 6.30 p.m. I immediately feel anxious and feel acutely aware of the adolescent who is at my side in the kitchen and a female staff member who is staring at Carla and Natalia with an extremely concerned expression on her face. "OK" I say, and stand up to walk out of the kitchen, away from the on-looking adolescent. As they follow, I say, "So the surgery shuts at half past six and you need to get there to collect your medication?" feeling anxious as

> I visualize the consequences of her not making it on time. "You'd better leave Natalia with me until you get back." She passes Natalia over to me with a warm bottle of milk and says "thank-you" before turning to walk quickly along the corridor and out of the building.

Such a response had been enhanced by my own developing internal capacity for reflection. My engagement with weekly work discussion seminars, the primary task of which were to facilitate in its members an increased capacity to observe, understand, and act, had modelled a regular, reflective thinking space in which I was able to stand back and reconsider experience in the workplace from a fresh perspective. In this case example, my own capacity to tolerate and think about other people's anxiety has started to develop. I had begun to internalize the model presented by the regular work discussion seminar.

Thinking back, I remember vividly literally being left "holding the baby" and the intense quality of the panic that Carla had powerfully projected into me. Freud (1895d) and Klein (1946) associated the term "projection" with a process in which parts of the self and certain states of mind are located in another. At this moment, Carla projects her own lack of responsibility onto her absent, unreliable partner in her statement, "he is just leaving us on our own and taking no responsibility"—evacuating, perhaps, the internal discomfort aroused by her partner's unreliability and an accompanying limited capacity for containment (Bion, 1962a). Bion likened containment to the function of the mother whose ability to receive and understand the emotional states of her baby makes them more bearable. Carla's mental illness and current state of high anxiety would be likely to impact adversely upon her capacity to contain at this moment.

I felt relief as she left me holding her daughter but was able to think about and process what had happened and therefore provide some containment for Carla's anxiety and actual physical care to Natalia in the absence of her mother. I had maintained a capacity for reasonably clear thinking and thus minimized the impingement of this mini crisis on the other work tasks of the centre. When Carla returned from the surgery, she appeared more relaxed. She had been able to collect her prescription, and both she and Natalia were pleased to be reunited. I expressed my pleasure that she had been able to get her medication and reassured her that Natalia had been fine in her absence. I felt satisfied that I had offered a helpful and supportive response.

Dysfunction, splitting, and "bizarre objects" in the family assessment task

Three and a half months later I worked with the Smith family, who had been admitted to the centre for a three-month comprehensive residential family assessment. The family comprised Margaret, mother, aged 19, with a mild learning disability, Anthony, father, aged 25, diagnosed with a personality disorder and a history of drug and alcohol misuse, and their 8-month-old son, James. James had received a non-accidental injury in his 6th month, allegedly from his father in the presence of his mother. Both parents had themselves grown up in care and had experienced disrupted and deprived childhoods. The following is a description of work I undertook with this family in the first month of their time at the centre.

> Anthony answered the door, looked at me and slightly raised his eyebrows before turning quickly to walk back down the corridor. I said "Hi" and could see James heading towards me in a square-shaped baby walker full of buttons with pictures, squeakers, tunes, and a bright red plastic telephone. . . . I walked into the sitting room, where Margaret was sitting watching the television, which had images of violent conflict in the Middle East blaring out rather loudly. She looked at me and made half an attempt to acknowledge my presence before refocusing on the television. James reappeared in his walker, whizzing around the room excitedly, at the same time looking at each of us.

My immediate sense of feeling unwelcome often characterized time spent with this family. Baby James in his self-contained "cell" of self-provision also appeared unwelcome in the minds of his often otherwise engaged or absent parents. My own sense of being unwelcome may have been associated with an unconscious identification with James in his lonely self-providing state or linked to percolating projective processes within the family.

> James continued to whiz around the room in his walker, seeming happy and contented until he bumped into his mother's foot. Margaret responded by gently kicking the walker away from her, complaining, "Ouch! That was my toe." James soon began to protest and grizzle. . . . This was accompanied by a desperate stare at his mother, who ignored him and continued to focus on the pages of the open magazine on her lap. Anthony listened intently to his

mobile phone. I felt increasingly anxious about the silence and their lack of interest in or preoccupation with James.

James's object-seeking behaviour may have connected with the cycle of neglect within this dysfunctional family unit. He really has become a nuisance in the same way that my presence as observer and assessor is a nuisance to his parents. My own experience of rejection, of feeling ignored, and of being an unwanted burden may have been a reflection of James's experience.

Mother and father's own experiences of deprived and institutionalized parenting probably failed to provide them with the necessary psychological and social capacities to manage and negotiate family life. A number of studies have investigated the intergenerational transmission of abuse, including Main and Goldwyn (1984), who were able to predict mother's rejection of her own infant from accounts of her experiences of her own mother as rejecting. Lyons-Ruth and Block (1996) noted that a history of physical abuse was associated with increased hostile and intrusive behaviour towards the infant, increased negative affect by the infant, and a decreased tendency to report trauma-related symptoms. In thinking about why parents tend to repeat abusive patterns, Egeland and Susman-Stillman (1996) hypothesized that it is dissociative processes that account for the transmission of maltreatment. Both Margaret and Anthony displayed dissociative, avoidant qualities during this piece of assessment work.

Bion (1962a) provides a psychoanalytic account of these phenomena. He describes pathological forms of development in which the experience of reality is felt primarily as persecution. This arouses violent hatred and consequent fragmentation of all experience of reality, external and internal. There is then no "tidy split" between an ideal and a bad object or objects; instead, the object is perceived as being split into tiny bits, each containing a minute and violently hostile part of the ego. These "bizarre objects" damage the ego through their persecutory nature and the painful mutilation of the perceptual apparatus (Segal, 1964). The introjection of institutional or "bizarre objects" by both parents as a consequence of disrupted and deprived childhood experiences appears to have impacted upon their ability to perform the containment or reverie functions of parenting. The result is a transgenerational re-enactment of neglectful patterns of parenting.

Margaret may have been presenting James with a projective-identification-rejecting object (Bion, 1962a). He, then, "reintrojects, not a fear of dying made tolerable, but a nameless dread" (Bion, 1962a, p. 116). The experience of repeated recurrence of this projective failure leads to the formation of an internal object that destroys meaning and leaves the subject in a mysterious meaningless world. The stripping of meaning by such an internal object gives rise to a superego that issues meaningless commands about behaviour (Hinshelwood, 1998). On this basis, James's experience of being parented may sadly mirror that of his own parents and fail to equip him with the necessary psychological and social function to grow, develop, and mature in a sophisticated manner.

These theoretical ideas can, however, lead one to premature diagnostic conclusions or hypotheses based on limited evidence, unless they are linked to emotionally engaged observation of oneself at work. It was the development of my own emotional engagement and capacity for close observation and reflection that attendance at work discussion seminars enhanced. There are few opportunities for reflection in a task-centred institution like the one described, and it was invaluable to be able to present often frustrating and overwhelming assessment work to a small group of colleagues whose observations, associations, and reflections generated fresh ideas and often painful yet productive self-reflection. I could return to the work feeling inspired and equipped with a clearer lens through which to view my task with children and families.

A month later I observed the family again. Two weeks prior to this, the parents had separated, and Anthony was no longer part of the assessment.

> Margaret picked up a tub of Sudocream after moving a box of toys that James had become quite fascinated with, repeatedly dipping his hand in and trying to pull out one toy at a time. She liberally rubbed cream into his bottom, which turned bright white, and then embarked upon a marathon attempt to put a nappy on him. He wriggled and squirmed, making it very difficult for Margaret to fasten the nappy. Almost as soon as she had got one part done, he would roll over, and the nappy would come off once again. This happened on at least two or three occasions before Margaret finally was able to fasten both parts of the nappy effectively. James looked as if he was thriving on what appeared to be a well-rehearsed routine, while Margaret patiently struggled to settle James into a position in which his nappy could be fastened but did not engage in the potential play and fun at all.

Discussion of this work in a seminar made me aware of a hitherto unconscious change in my attitude towards James and his mother. In the previous assessment work with both parents, I had tended towards viewing father, Anthony, as bad, and mother, Margaret, as good. With Anthony's departure and Margaret now being more precisely assessed in his absence, I had begun to be able to notice some of the negative or poor parenting in Margaret. This type of splitting, often unconscious, is characteristic of Klein's (1946) paranoid–schizoid position. This phenomenon is pervasive and widespread in work with deprived and damaged children and families and can lead to poor practice and tensions within and between staff members and teams. A conscious awareness of the impact of splitting can facilitate healthier and more mature and functional modes of operating and providing services. The meta position provided by the work discussion seminar, the viewing of events from a fresh, slightly distant position, allowed me to see the part I played in interactions with peers and service users and generated a different level of conscious awareness.

Seminar group members expressed consistent concern about the precise nature of my role as family assessment worker. Was I there simply to assess, or did I have a duty not only to assess but also to provide encouragement and support to the families I was working with?

I had remained silent during the aforementioned routine of nappy changing, offering no practical encouragement, support, or celebration of achievement when Margaret finally succeeded in getting the nappy on James. I felt critical of Margaret's reluctance or inability to interact playfully with James, offering no reinforcement of positives or running commentary on what I was observing. Margaret's avoidant qualities and struggle to multi-task or "whole object" relate may have served to reinforce and perpetuate my overemphasis on assessment and almost complete lack of support and encouragement in my attitude to her.

I came to see that Margaret's relationships had a functional rather than emotionally alive quality. Margaret, in the nappy-changing ritual above, has a well-developed ability to focus on one part of James' care at a time. This "part-object" care-giving and manner of relating may have its roots in her own experience of being parented. Such disconnectedness may, in turn, have exacerbated my own tendency towards silent, non-interventionist assessment rather than active family support. On reflection there was also likely to have been a part of me, my own valency (Bion, 1962a), that influenced my maintaining such a safe or defensive distance. Aspects of my own avoidant qualities may well have been in unconscious identification with those of Margaret. Later in the same observation:

> Margaret was out of the room at this point. James dropped his beaker on the duvet by his side and stretched to reach for a small toy Dalmatian, which he put on his lap. He soon began to search for his beaker and quickly located it with his hand, gripping the yellow spout and lifting it towards his face. The beaker was half-empty, so all his attempts to suck and drink were unsuccessful because he was unable to achieve the necessary angle to allow the juice to flow. He peered at the beaker and tried and tried to tip the juice into this mouth using one hand on the handle. He persevered with different variations of holding the spout and tipping, holding one handle and tipping, and holding the other and tipping, occasionally dropping the beaker before lifting it up and trying again. This fascinating display continued for what seemed like a few minutes before Margaret returned to the room.
>
> On her arrival, James began to protest and dropped the beaker on the duvet, picking it back up for one last attempt. Oblivious to his excruciating lack of success to get a drink, Margaret began to play with another toy Dalmatian that had what looked like a dummy in its mouth and which barked when this was taken out.

Here Margaret turns to the toy dog while overlooking the needs of James. I again think critical thoughts about her parenting capacity rather than saying something to help her such as, "I think he would like a drink. While you were out he's been trying to drink from his beaker." Perhaps my own over-identification with James had led to my empathy being located with him rather than with Margaret, who had, after all, been left in the lone carer role. Alternatively, I could have chosen to help James with his beaker in Margaret's absence, role-modelling good child care but perhaps compromising or blurring my role of assessment worker. In family assessment work the tendency to overly identify with one family member is, perhaps, inevitable. My ongoing attendance at work discussion seminars provided an increased awareness of these complex processes and encouraged this level of self-reflection.

Within Margaret there did not appear to be a very developed concept that the other person is relating to her. This lack of meaningful connections led to a lack of responsiveness to cues for intervention. A form of mis-steps in the relational dance then ensued. Such factors could impact upon the nature of Margaret and James's attachment as well as the emotional experience of assessing and observing their relationship.

An increasing awareness of unconscious processes and influences within and between was beginning to emerge for me. This "added dimension" to my capacity to think about and process my own emotional experience alongside the emotional experience of those I was observing generated increased space for developing my assessment work. I was acting and intervening and becoming more aware that doing nothing is also an intervention.

Role clarification and primary task definition in adolescent assessment work: or why is emotionality numbed?

Five months later I presented an account of my experience in a staff meeting to the work discussion seminar. The emotional challenge of working in a short-term assessment centre emerged alongside the pain of undertaking assessment as opposed to more reparative tasks.

> As I had been in the admissions meeting the previous day, I began to discuss the details of a 13-year-old girl who had just been admitted to the centre. She arrived after staying one night in foster care, following a breakdown in her relationship with her mother. Just as I was describing the main content of yesterday's admissions meeting, I noticed one or two people staring out of the window. Initially I thought they were just not listening, but I soon realized that something was going on outside. I stopped talking, and one of them said that the police had just pulled up outside. I continued discussing the young person until a colleague popped her head into the room and announced that the police were here to arrest the young person we were discussing! I suggested to the other deputy that we would need to provide an appropriate adult to accompany her to the police station, because she was only 13.

An overwhelming feeling of despair in this meeting was identified through exploration in the work discussion seminar. The impotence of the staff team attempting to provide care for this young person was hard to bear alongside the knowledge that her predicament could be talked about but not in any way controlled. The work task with this and many of the other young people seemed to border on the impossible.

Rice (1963) defined "primary task" as the task an organization must perform if it is to survive. On this basis the dual primary tasks of the family resource centre are to perform family assessment and adolescent assessment work. Task definition within the helping professions is notoriously difficult, and within the assessment centre there was a consistent need for clarity of task with each individual young person and family. Clarifying the task of the work with this young person was impossible at this stage as a consequence partly of circumstances but also of poor information exchange. The lack of clarity generated high levels of anxiety and a prevailing lack of hope. It was easier to think and act in a task-focused way than in a manner that may have brought the thinking and action of the staff team closer to a consideration of the emotional experience of the young person.

The task of the centre is to assess, not to do therapeutic work. Miller and Rice (1967) developed the idea of open systems theory. Using this model, the centre's output is assessment of teenagers and their families. The "how" of the performance of this task was the recurring theme in my work discussion seminar. What balance should there be between observing and monitoring with the assessment function and helping or training in parenting? What is the influence of this balance or the likely influence on the morale and emotional experience of staff? Low morale is commonplace within local authority resources, which have a tendency towards very task-centred, crisis-led ways of working. An institutional denial or naiveté about the emotional content of the work and the influence of unconscious processes seemed prevalent in my own place of work. My own experience was that I frequently felt I learnt and spoke one language in the work discussion context but actually adopted and spoke another in my work environment. This experience may well have reflected my own personal development at the time. The split-off experience could have been integrated in a different way. I may have been able to work towards sharing some of the fresh ideas and thoughts aroused in work discussion with colleagues in a thoughtful, sensitive manner. In fact, what happened seemed to be that I took on too much of the collective despair at the expense, perhaps, of holding and representing the hopefulness that can accompany creative thinking and discussion.

My consistent experience tended to be of feeling frustrated at the overemphasis in team discussions on symptoms and behaviours.

Concrete events were repeatedly discussed at the expense of questioning and consideration of why such behaviours and events occur and how we might influence change. Powerful institutional defences seemed to be in place that led to a numbing of emotionality and absence of thinking.

For example, the management team introduced a new written format for daily shift reviews that included in it the question, "How did it feel to work with this teenager/family?" The lack of consultation within the process led to the new system's eventual sabotage by the team. However, during the trial stages I remember feeling so exasperated at everyone's reluctance, unwillingness, or resistance to engage with this exploration of emotion that I responded cuttingly to one staff member who used the word "fine" to describe their feelings by saying that this was a texture, not a feeling. Clearly this sort of remark did not help to create the atmosphere of safety and trust necessary for people to begin to be open and honest about their emotional experience at work.

In team meetings I tended to feel a whole host of powerful emotions, from despair, anger, and sadness to impotence, helplessness, and uselessness. I often occupied an advocate-type role for young people, encouraging my colleagues to think about the needs of the young people and the reasons why they behaved and felt the way they did. Clearly aspects of my experience reflected unconscious projective and identificatory processes that are inherent aspects of this type of work setting. The arousal of aspects of my own unresolved emotional experience will also have played a part.

Staff meetings had a tendency to become septic tanks serving some kind of containment function. I would find myself asking contentious questions at the same time as striving to identify needs in the knowledge that we might realistically only go part of the way to meeting them.

> The keyworker of a 13-year-old girl who had been admitted the previous week began to update and outline to the team the nature of her family circumstances and admission, placing a lot of emphasis on what had not happened and what had not been done. . . . Then followed in-depth discussion of her persistent overnight absconding since admission and her intoxication and bad behaviour the previous evening. Feeling irritated that nobody appeared to be advocating on her behalf, I asked the team what we were going to do about yesterday's events and what services we felt

> we could provide to this young person. I highlighted that we had two keyworkers in the room who are working with her. . . . The keyworkers then described the social worker's inactivity, and the discussion left me irritated, as it seemed nobody really wanted to take much responsibility or initiative.

In this typical scenario in my role of duty manager I became embroiled in the professional dynamics surrounding the life of a classically deprived, unsocial "looked-after" teenager. The dynamic of blame projected onto an inactive, unreliable social worker by the keyworker may mirror aspects of the parental relationship within the child's family of origin. At the same time as the child struggles to take any responsibility for investing in her new temporary home and relationships, so, too, do members of the professional network struggle to take responsibility for performing their professional tasks and functions.

My own irritation may have as one of its sources the child's own fury and disorientation. This may then trickle through the layers of containment in the boundaries or semi-permeable membranes surrounding the child. In the absence of parents, the corporate parenting of the staff team provides the initial layer of such a membrane. In the duty manager's role I performed the task of paternal containment by providing a secondary semi-permeable membrane. This type of boundary management is described in detail by Miller and Rice (1967). The skill and challenge for anyone occupying this type of role is to attempt to maintain some capacity for thinking. Within such thinking space, one can begin to consider the numerous complex conscious and unconscious processes in operation. An ability to process the gut instinct or emotion allows it to be used as a type of diagnostic tool. This is skilled work, requiring a sophisticated level of self-awareness and capacity to share complex ideas in a non-threatening and palatable manner. For me, this process was modelled and enhanced through committed attendance at work discussion.

That is how my feelings of irritation came to serve as fuel for thought and ideas of practical interventions and possible solutions rather than as tinder for irrational, angry, critical reactions targeted at the "useless" staff members who did not appear to care. When I could maintain thinking space from a boundary position, hopefully I provided some containment and encouragement to those leaving the discussion to work directly with the young person.

The added dimension: a greater capacity to track emotionality

The most consistent theme that emerged for me in the work discussion was the question of just what, precisely, was the aim of the assessment work of the centre and how I, as a practitioner, contributed to this task. For me, this process was both fascinating yet painful. Was I really simply policing these young people and families, gathering hard evidence to eventually present to court? Or did I have a responsibility to perform a family-support and parenting development type of function?

Regular discussion and analysis of the "unconscious at work" in the work discussion seminar generated a great deal of self-examination and of learning about inter- and intra-psychic processes from a psychoanalytic perspective. The extent to which my own interventions were influenced by unconscious pressures became more and more apparent, and this led to the development of an increased capacity to think and pay attention to the invisible distortions of the assessment work of the centre.

Feeling more in touch with my own experience enabled me not only to self-monitor and more accurately assess but also to tune in to and track what I would describe as the emotionality of those with whom I was working. Observational skills helped me to retain information of events from memory and to attend to fine detail. A developing awareness of the emotional experience of transference and countertransference feelings also enhanced my ability to think and act more creatively in the face of what was very challenging work.

My functioning within the role of family assessment worker was enhanced over time by actively thinking about finding a balance between pure observation and assessment and family support and encouragement. I was increasingly able to hold in mind individuals and whole families, at the same time as raising questions and generating multiple ideas to consider. I was more able to think about unconscious influences at the same time as providing actual support and grounded interventions, and I began to be able to consider the internal worlds of children and family members and to link experiences of past, present, and future.

PART III

INTERNATIONAL CONTRIBUTIONS

CHAPTER EIGHT

"Sibonye is stuck . . .": the work discussion model adapted to South African conditions

Sheila Miller

"Sibonye is stuck", said his crèche principal, and she went on to add that she meant this literally, as he "spends all his time in the 'block area'", playing rather mechanically with blocks and small vehicles, and he simply cannot be persuaded to take part in any other activities. At mealtimes, she said, he ate voraciously, never seeming satisfied. The only place other than the block area that he would go to was the classroom of a teacher of an older group of children. She let him sit close to her while she worked and, in the eyes of the rest of the staff, was "spoiling" him. Tandi, the principal, an experienced and calm person, conveyed a sense of deadlock. This 3-year old was obviously engendering desperation and despair. Her comments showed that she had genuine concern for the boy himself but was also worried about what it meant to other children that he was allowed to miss the story ring and other activities. The "problem" was affecting crèche routine and also causing staff tension between herself and the member of staff who was "spoiling" him. The staff had all been patient with him thus far, and now that the end of his first year was approaching, she felt that something needed to be done.

Behind this "problem" lies not pathology, but a tragedy. Sibonye's parents both died of AIDS—first his father, over a year before, and some months later his mother. The family had lived in a country adjoining South Africa. After losing their parents, Sibonye and his older sister were fostered by an uncle and aunt in Soweto, a township adjacent to Johannesburg. Although the family was stressed by the situation, being themselves bereaved as well as having taken on an enormous responsibility, the children were well and lovingly cared for. But Sibonye had remained, Tandi told us, very clingy at home and wanted to call his aunt "mother", which enraged his 9-year old sister, Boni, who would cry out desperately, "Don't you know our mother is dead?" Boni herself was often angry and hostile to her aunt, Pindi, and her teacher was worried that she was not performing to potential.

The setting in which this account was given was a "work discussion" group, led by my colleague, Lesley Caplan, a clinical psychologist, and me, a child and adolescent psychotherapist. The group members were the director, senior trainers, supervisors, and some crèche principals belonging to an organization that runs many excellent crèches in Soweto. Creches in this area are similar to British preschool nurseries. They cater for children from 2 to 6 but are structured like schools, with the workers being known as teachers. The organization invests a great deal of time, effort, and financial support in the training of their staff, so that child care and the content of activities provided are of a high standard. Their training is focused on an understanding of good physical and educative child care but with very little attention to emotional development. Principals and teachers, like the director, trainers, and supervisors, have an exceedingly busy routine, with very little time for quiet reflection and discussion. The principal, in addition to strenuous administrative duties, often has to deal with the personal problems of parents and staff members, as well as the behavioural and emotional development of the children.

The "work discussion" meeting described was part of a pilot project to explore whether the opportunity for supervisors, trainers, and crèche staff to share their pressing work problems, with the assistance of outside consultants, would add a useful dimension to their work. My colleague and I decided to use the Tavistock work discussion model that had in the 1970s been introduced for staff by various other agencies, among them the Camden Young Families project and several Camden children's homes. The Young Families centres catered for under-five children whose families were experiencing difficulties, and most of the children had suffered deprivation and neglect. The work discussions were led by Tavistock staff child psychotherapists, but the way of working had to be adapted, bearing in mind that these meetings differed from the Observational Studies Course seminars in many respects: the groups were larger than the five-person seminars, and all participants were employed in the same setting, which made them feel very vulnerable when exposing how they worked. From my own experience in a Young Family Centre and various Children's Homes I knew that written observations were unlikely to come easily to the crèche workers, so we decided to depend on verbal description. Although work discussions are usually led by one person, we decided in this instance to work jointly, as we felt we needed mutual support in undertaking such a new venture .We were, in fact, able to complement one another. We shared devotion to a psychoanalytic perspective and knowledge of child development. I had substantial experience of leading work discussions in various London settings, but she understood South African conditions. She understood the model but had not previously used it. I think this made her more open to adaptation and that the teachers were good observers. Their training had been geared towards achieving succinct formal description, and they were surprised that we were looking for a free reflective mode of dialogue based on detailed observation. We found that the teachers could give good descriptions of the children and parents, but they were unused to discussing in detail the implications of what they saw and heard and, in particular, of what they felt. We also realized very soon that flexibility was important and that we had to take account of local circumstances and what the group members felt they needed.

Sibonye's plight was an example of the extreme and tragic nature of some of the problems that confronted staff. Other cases raised ranged from symptoms like separation anxiety and biting, which occur in all settings where young children are cared for, to concerns about precociously sexual behaviour, which might indicate abuse or might arise from other causes. But what was most striking was the impact on staff and children of the violence that occurs daily in Soweto and, indeed, in Johannesburg and many other areas of South Africa. As well as dealing with traumatic occurrences that impinge on the work of the crèches, it was clear that staff members were also constantly stressed by traumas that touched their personal lives and their emotions. In the space of one meeting, incidents mentioned included the recent murder of the husband of one of the crèche teachers, the fact that a trainer present had recently lost her husband in tragic circumstances and had herself been shot and wounded in an earlier incident, while another trainer voiced her concern about a friend whose home-loving and well-adjusted young son had been killed in a senseless street fight. The course of the discussion revealed the complexities of dealing with the practical and emotional levels of personal shock and distress in the lives of the children and in the community at large.

Freeing the group to speak

To return to Sibonye, when the group had heard about the death of his parents and how he and his sister had been alone with their ill mother for many months and then remained in the house in the care of a relative while she was in hospital until her death, there was a deep silence. It was a long time until anyone felt able to speak. (In retrospect, we thought that this was a mirroring of the paralysis experienced by Sibonye himself in the wake of his cumulative trauma.) We spent some time asking for more information: some details about exactly what was happening at school and at home. We also asked for some suggestions from the group. The group members were diffident, and we felt under pressure to provide a solution. When one of us commented on the effect the details of the history was having on the group, this seemed to free people to talk. Comments were made that showed that as well as the deaths, there were many other stressors in the situation. We drew these together, pointing out that the children had suffered multiple trauma and that, as well as losing both their parents, the long illness of their mother had severely curtailed their ordinary activities and opportunities for development. Furthermore, they had been subjected to tremendous disruption and had to accommodate to living in a new family and in urban surroundings that were very different from their rural home village.

The group found it useful when we commented that numbness and lethargy are common in the early stages of bereavement but that these can be much prolonged where there has been cumulative trauma. In thinking about what the children might have understood of the experience, it also emerged that no one had actually talked to them about the bereavement or about their parents' illness. There was discussion about whether this would be useful or whether it was better for them to forget about it. I felt able to say emphatically that they needed the opportunity to talk about their experiences and what they knew and understood of what had happened. They might need information as well as sympathy. Nevertheless I also felt it important to enquire about whether open discussion would conflict with cultural tradition. It seemed that this was not the case in this family, although in some areas death would only be whispered about to children when asleep. As often happens, however, the adults had been preoccupied with practical matters as well as the anxiety of how to speak to the children about the tragic circumstances. This work was done before HIV AIDS had reached epidemic proportions, and little information and training was available to workers. We commented on the difficulty of discussing AIDS and whether the particular fears and the sexual implications of AIDS might have made it even more difficult to talk to the children. We all shared a sense of great relief when, following a question, we were told that tests had been done and that the children were HIV-negative. We touched on how difficult it can be for adults to discuss painful topics with children and how this can relate to one's own distressing experiences. We spoke also of the strains that were involved for the foster family, who had several children of their own. Though some discussion followed, the mood remained sombre, but this was relieved a bit when my colleague commented on this and linked it again to the material we had been discussing.

The principal indicated that she and her staff needed help but also wanted some feedback for the foster-parents. On hearing more about the foster-mother, it seemed clear that she and her husband would be able to talk to the children, but that she might need some discussion to prepare her for the task. My colleague offered to provide a limited number of sessions that would focus on her own stress and on her dealings with the children. As it was likely that the little boy did not himself know consciously why he was so troubled and might well find it difficult to articulate this, we suggested that someone whom he knew well in the school might spend time with him and encourage him to do some free and undirected drawing, to see if either the drawings or his description of them would give any clue to his state of mind. The matter of his clinging to the teacher who was "spoiling" him was discussed in the light of the regression that is usually seen in bereaved children and the possibility that, following the death of his mother, he might fear leaving the side of caring adults in case they, too, might disappear. We also explored whether he was causing any disruption in the class, but it seemed he just sat quietly. When considering the "greedy" eating, one of the group members wondered whether there had been a scarcity of food during mother's illness, which was a possibility even though the children had not been malnourished on arrival. It was also possible that it was a concrete way of filling an empty mental space or a reminder of an early good feeding experience that he was trying to hold on to. These points were speculative but were made in an attempt to postulate a view on the boy's internal state. We also hoped to encourage the idea that experience and behaviour have internal correlates. With time it might be possible to talk about unconscious phantasy.

The importance of ritual was touched on, and group members wondered whether the children would be taken back to their hometown in the approaching Christmas holiday and whether it would be important to visit their parents' graves. This led to further discussion about bereavement, and there were some questions about the length of normal mourning processes, the implication being that a year was a long period for such an acute response. We replied, stressing that the grief process could be prolonged but that if it continued for another six months without alleviation, one might have to think about a referral to a children's clinic. We were left feeling that our suggestions seemed rather paltry in the face of the enormity of the problem posed.

At the following meeting, the principal, Tandi, showed us some drawings done by Sibonye in her presence. At first sight they were meaningless scribbles, but she explained that the vague circle in the middle was a chair and that Sibonye, pointing to it, had said something about "mama"; the squiggle next to it was his sister, and somewhere on the periphery were some cars.

This was a dramatic illustration of the centrality of his mother in his thoughts, as he had not been told what to draw. Tandi said she had been reluctant to ask him if he meant his biological or foster-mother, but the drawing helped to convince her that the loss of his mother still preoccupied him. Group members initially seemed sceptical about whether any of this was pertinent but did become interested. One member puzzled over the meaning of the vehicles, wondering whether they stood for his wish to go back to his old home in the hope of finding his mother, or whether they were related to his memory of coming to Soweto by car. Tandi said the foster-mother had been talking to the children about their parents and had found it less difficult than she had expected.

The family were going to spend the Christmas holidays in the children's home country and were wondering how the children would react to the experience. The counselling sessions for the foster-mother had not yet taken place, but as we were told that she was still very stressed, an appointment was arranged. We used a portion of the rest of that session to draw together in a more formal way some information on the stages of bereavement in children.

At the following meeting, which took place some four weeks later, after the Christmas holidays, Tandi told us that the foster-mother had found a considerable improvement in both children. Boni was now much less hostile to her and more tolerant of Sibonye's wish to call their aunt "mama". Pindi had a scarf that had belonged to the children's mother, and Boni now wanted her aunt to wear it. Boni's teacher had reported that there had been an improvement in her schoolwork. By the end of term, Sibonye had begun to venture out of the block area and had maintained the improvement in the new term. The family had spent the Christmas period near the children's old home, and although the holiday had been successful, to the parents' surprise both children had been pleased to return to their Soweto home. Tandi said that it had been helpful to her to see Sibonye's relationship to the other teacher as part of the bereavement process rather than as spoiling.

We could all acknowledge that a definite shift had taken place, but it was also important to point out that the mourning process is not a finite one, and that there might be a repetition of the same symptoms or the occurrence of other reactions. Therefore some time was spent alerting Tandi about this possibility by referring to the importance of anniversaries and other triggers that might re-evoke the traumatic memories.

I shall describe now the reasoning that informed the way we went about addressing this problem. On first hearing the account of Sibonye's behaviour, before the history was mentioned, many possibilities came to mind, such as separation anxiety, depression, trauma, or abuse. Tandi's tone and the length of time the symptoms had persisted suggested that there was something seriously amiss, and I found myself thinking that this case needed to be referred for an assessment. When the loss of both parents and all the other traumatic elements were revealed, this thought persisted, but I reminded myself silently of the danger of dealing with anxiety by sending the problem elsewhere. As the discussion continued and the group members showed that they had grasped the nub of the problem, both my colleague and I sensed that there was much that could be done by those in the child's familiar surroundings.

Given the scarcity of therapy provision that could be accessed by this family, it seemed sensible to address the problem by using the resources of the family and the crèche. For a number of reasons this was, in fact, the method of choice and not just of expedience. Breaking the news about death or giving information about the circumstances is always best done by adults who know the children well and have a sympathetic relation to them. This also has the advantage of ensuring a space for the children to talk freely in the family about the tragic events. It was, however, important to bear in mind the question of whether these foster-parents could manage the task, and to try to judge whether Tandi, who had to mediate by passing on the information to them, felt enough confidence in the suggestion to do so successfully. Furthermore, it was necessary to try to involve the group in evolving the strategy and to address any anxieties or intellectual doubts they might have about it. Comments passed by group members (some of whom knew Pindi well) and confirmed by Tandi gave the impression that, although stressed, she had considerable strength. The decision to offer Pindi some counselling sessions was based on my colleague's sense from what we had heard that this would need to be only a short-term intervention and could be made within the context of the work. Where family support is available professionally, the facilitators of a work discussion group would not offer individual interventions, but we thought it justified as receiving other help was highly unlikely. This proved to be correct, but it would not be either practical or desirable for the consultation/work discussion to become a clinical service. Probably, though, some leeway would always be needed to deal with some individual difficulties outside the group (Irvine, 1959). This is certainly the case until more local provision is available. We thought that a possible solution might be to organize a therapeutic service parallel to the work discussions, which could accept and work with referrals of adults and children.

The suggestion that someone in the crèche should let Sibonye do some undirected drawing was based on the hope that this might help him make a more direct contact than was possible in either the close but regressed relationship he had made with the caring teacher who tended to pet him, or in the cut-off stance he maintained when "stuck" in the block area. The speed with which he addressed what most preoccupied him surprised us. Although very little was said to him, it seems that the serious attention of an adult really trying to receive his communication made him feel understood and contained some of his unbearable feelings (Bion, 1962a). The question arises as to whether it is appropriate to scrutinize drawings in a school setting in the same way as one might do in a contained therapy space. The groups are aimed at fostering an awareness of internal processes and not at teaching an interpretative technique, so it is important to stress the speculative nature of any comment and the fact that definitive conclusions should not be based on such evidence.

I do not consider that a fundamental therapeutic change has been effected by the strategy employed. The suggestions formulated in the group and carried out by family and crèche staff have provided conditions that facilitate normal mourning processes. One cannot be complacent about the children's long-term development, but I trust the intervention will also alert the family to the importance of monitoring their progress.

The work discussion group

The example of Sibonye and his family, which occupied a part of each meeting, has been quoted at length to illustrate one of the possible functions of such a group, but also to serve as a focus for discussing the professional and ethical implications of this way of working. The account, though accurate in itself, gives an oversimplified picture of the much richer but more complicated and at times troubled experience of the four group meetings that comprised this pilot scheme. There were some discussions about the extent to which sexual matters can be discussed with children in African families, and there were allusions to changes in custom pertaining to graveside ritual, which could not be developed in the time available. These allusions hinted at considerable problems around what traditional beliefs and customs should be retained, and at a struggle to sort out what is a justifiable evolution and accommodation to modern life and what is a denial of cultural heritage. This is, of course, not restricted to South African life, but we hoped that perhaps over time there might be space to elucidate the particular elements that affect daily life in the area we were working in. As white psychologists and psychotherapists, we were aware that issues of race and culture were bound to have a bearing on the course of the work. This particular organization has a long history of good working relationships between black and white workers, though there must inevitably be complexities connected to race and personality that would affect such a group and their relationships to the consultants. In our contact with this group it seemed that what was more significant were the differences between the staff's way of approaching problems and our attempts to do so.

When in the third meeting there was a particularly sticky patch, some group members were fortunately able to air their disappointment at the way we had addressed the problems they had brought, though they clearly did not find it easy to do so. They let us know that they had expected more directive advice on how to manage children's difficulties but that, more urgently, they needed help in dealing with the personal problems of parents and crèche staff members for whom they were often the only resource. At that point, although it was clear that some good work had been done in connection with Sibonye and we had experienced the first two meetings positively, we became rather discouraged about whether we were able to offer what was needed.

Reviewing the contract

On reflection, we realized that although our original proposal had been accepted by the group, there had been—as is not unusual in consultation work—a discrepancy between the expectations they had of the meetings and what we thought we had outlined. At a rational level—and justifiably so—they had hoped for didactic "input" as well as expert advice on how to handle difficulties and had not anticipated that we were expecting to draw on their own expertise. At a less rational level there was perhaps the usual hope we all have that someone can solve problems swiftly and effortlessly and the disappointment and disillusionment that follows when this does not happen. Also pertinent is the fact that when a group has such high expectations, there is usually in parallel a feeling that much is being withheld by the so-called "experts" and a consequent undervaluing of their own experience and wisdom. Perhaps, also, they needed to convey their own repeated experience of being expected to supply solutions they considered to be beyond their capabilities.

By consensus, the following meeting started with a review, partly to address the dissatisfaction that had been voiced but also because it was the last meeting of the pilot phase, and we needed to know whether the organization wished us to continue the seminars. Several suggestions were made that were felt to be more useful—reading case studies in journals or formal lectures—and again the urgency of work with adults was stressed. All members of the crèche staff frequently had to deal with parents' distress and were also called upon for advice about children's behaviour and other parenting issues. They were also often upset by parents' and carers' inadequate care of children and were interested to hear a point of view that tried to understand the circumstances rather than being judgemental. The principal had to deal with the—often very acute—distress of the crèche staff. We indicated that we had no objection to difficulties in their dealings with parents and colleagues being raised but realized that it was essential for us to explain better how we saw the task. As mentioned earlier, we were in effect trying to introduce a model that posited an internal world and emphasized the importance of containment and reflection. By implication, we were suggesting that these concepts are applicable to children and adults, but with hindsight it seems to me that we did not stress enough the overlaps between the infant/child and the adult world.

We spoke at some length of our beliefs that by thinking together and pooling our mental resources, a way of dealing with problems could be evolved. We acknowledged our training and experience but also expressed our view that the group members tended to underestimate their own experience and capacity. As mentioned, during this meeting Tandi gave her feedback on Sibonye's family and expressed her opinion that the way the problem had been addressed had definitely worked in this case.

The anxiety and urgency about work with staff was illustrated when the matter was raised of Viccy, a staff member whose husband had recently been killed in front of her and their children in an act of criminal violence. The director put a formal question about what could be fairly expected from Viccy in her state of grief. There were serious implications for staffing if she were not able to fulfil her duties. It was obvious that the director herself was shocked by the personal tragedy of Viccy, whom she knows well. She had helped with the practical arrangements, made inquiries about trauma debriefing, and described graphically with a sense of outrage the legal hassle that was involved for the bereaved family. In talking, she seemed suddenly touched with how all this "busyness", though essential, was also a way of coping with the horror of the incident itself and with the general state of violence in the community. On our enquiring further, it emerged from the comments of other staff members that Viccy was coping at present, especially as the principal of her crèche had a very good personal relationship with her.

We discussed the fact that response to shock and response to bereavement, though showing common features, also differed in individuals, and my colleague pointed out that therefore some people might need to withdraw, while others might find work—particularly work with children—to be therapeutic. The group took this up, and discussion followed, weighing up whether or not Viccy needed relief from duties. The consensus seemed to be that she could manage but that the situation would need to be monitored. I argued that for Viccy, as for Sibonye, one might expect that there would be changes in her reaction over time, and I expanded on the way that seemingly unconnected and trivial incidents might trigger traumatic memories, causing reactions that could be misunderstood unless this was taken into account. My description included some specific examples of how the prolonged reaction to trauma and bereavement might cause difficulties in the work situation for adults if colleagues did not understand this.

At this point Cindy, one of the trainers, burst into tears, saying that this was true and that it resonated for her. She was so distressed that she had to leave the room. Someone followed to comfort her, and we all sat silently for a moment, and then people started to explain quietly that she had ongoing and past tragedies in her family. On her return, group members were very supportive towards her, but I was left feeling worried that my examples had been expressed too intensely and that we had not contained the meeting properly. My response was to ask her afterwards if she would like a referral to another therapist for some help, and she agreed that she would.

On resuming discussion of whether the groups should continue, there was firm support for this: the group members who had earlier expressed their disappointment now said they understood better what we were trying to achieve. We also now had a clearer idea of what might be helpful. We had assumed that problems concerning child development would be the most important area to address, but now knew that, at least for the next series of meetings, the group needed difficulties with adults to be addressed.

Boundary between task group and therapy group

When some days later I called to tell Cindy that I had found a suitable vacancy for an exploratory meeting, she said she would take up the offer but also added spontaneously and in a genuine way that she had felt much better after the meeting and that sharing her distress had been very helpful. Though this had worked out well, it is in such instances that the boundary between a task-oriented group and a therapeutic group becomes an issue. We are clear that a group of colleagues meeting in their work setting is not an appropriate membership for a therapeutic group, but we are aware that some of the issues that are raised for individuals will be similar to those that would arise and be dealt with in a therapeutic setting. The method of eliciting detailed information and encouraging careful observation puts the members of the group in touch with the pain and aggression of their clients in a way that is not encountered when abstraction and labelling are used. This can breach the defensive mechanisms usually employed, so that if interpretation cannot be used, other containing measures will need to be taken. A structured approach that requires a prepared and detailed presentation of problems is one way of providing containment. Another safeguard is to move flexibly between what one might term a didactic approach and a dialectic and reflective mode. At all times it must be borne in mind that the priority is training and that the group members are there as fully responsible adult professionals and not as patients or clients.

The pilot led to several series of work discussion meetings with staff members of crèches that were considered useful. In an informal evaluation the feedback was that the discussions, as well as being supportive, had resulted in a change of attitude. One member said that they now understood that children were not just naughty but that what they do has a meaning. Unfortunately funding difficulties in the organization prevented the work from continuing. However, the work discussion model, with adaptations to suit particular conditions, has been introduced into a number of other community projects and agencies.

This is supported and promoted by the development in Johannesburg and Cape Town of a Tavistock model observational studies course.

Conclusion

Introducing this model poses many challenges in addition to the problem of obtaining financial support. The fabric of South African families has been severely disrupted for decades by the laws and practices that promoted the migrant labour system, as well as by the other cruel impositions of apartheid. Currently the levels of violence impinge on daily living in a way that makes it very difficult to help children to feel secure. Added to this is the diversity of culture, languages, and child-rearing practices, which, though adding richness, also means that many traditions have to be taken into account in building up an understanding of what will be most useful for parents and professionals in bringing up a healthy new generation. From the discussions in the groups seen so far, it is clear that the distinction between an Afrocentric and a Eurocentric perspective is not a simple one. The issue is complicated by the usual difficulties of each generation deciding what aspects of family customs to retain and what aspects to change. A worker in one of the groups expressed her puzzlement in relation to mourning rituals, saying that her grandmother had placed a pot of beer on her grandfather's grave, and that this seemed foreign to her, but that placing flowers seemed a "white" practice, so that she felt unclear where she herself stood. It will clearly take time for norms to evolve that suit community life in a free society. There is, however, consensus about the importance of education and care for future generations. The work will have to proceed drawing on local models as well as overseas contributions, and with an openness to evaluation and learning from experience.

Note

My thanks to African Self-help for their permission to use the material and for what we learned from them. Thanks also to my colleagues Lesley Caplan, Lauren Gower, and Lillian Tombi Cingo.

CHAPTER NINE

Parenting a new institution

Simonetta M. G. Adamo, Serenella Adamo Serpieri, Paola Giusti, & Rita Tamajo Contarini

The Chance Project

The Chance Project is an initiative whose main purpose is the educational and social re-integration of a group of teenage drop-outs, aged between 14 and 16. It aims to enable these adolescents to obtain a school diploma by combining academic education, focused on the achievement of literacy, with the learning of social and practical skills. The range of activities is designed to re-instil a fundamental motivation to learn through an educational programme that is wide-ranging and personally meaningful, and through opportunities for developing cooperative skills.

Chance consists of three centres set up within schools in deprived areas of Naples—the historical centre and two outlying districts. Each centre has a coordinator, and there are also two head teachers, one of whom holds responsibility for the legal and administrative aspects, while the other coordinates the educational activities. Each year 80–90 children are involved, so over the nine-year period over 700 have passed through the project.

Children are recommended for inclusion by social services. Their lives have been marked by bereavement, abandonment, and disrupted primary relationships. The majority have an extremely restricted command of language; they display a tendency to impulsive action and little capacity to think. Their sense of identity is closely linked to their families, whose experiences and problems engulf their lives. Their families suffer from many problems: unemployment, poverty, physical and mental illness; additionally, many of the parents are involved in illegal activities or are part of organized crime (the "*Camorra*"); most are single-parent families due to the absence of the father, who is either in prison or has been killed in conflicts between rival gangs. The children's peer relationships are practically non-existent, and many of them have the duties and responsibilities of an adult. To a much greater extent than ordinary adolescents, they display an improbable combination of infantile fears and needs, together with pseudo-adult traits and behaviour.

The Project offers a favourable student–teacher ratio: 18 teachers, together with youth tutors and other specialists. A central role is also performed by the "social mothers". This term refers to a new and unusual professional role. These women all have children of their own; they began to work in the Project on a voluntary basis and now play a full part in the team, sharing all the in-service training opportunities. Their function (Adamo Serpieri & Giusti, 2007) is mainly that of welcoming the young people in the morning, preparing breakfast and lunch for them at school, and containing them in school when they are unable to stay in the classroom. We could say that the social mothers preside over all the intermediate spaces, both concretely and symbolically. They thus help to create a space between impulse and action, a "buffer" or "room for thought" (Bradley, 1991) in the physical structure of the school and in the children's experience. The role of the youth tutors has also evolved over the years. They organize the social activities of students, such as visits, trips, and summer camps, but also share in the running of the daily school routine.

However, it is the teachers who are at the centre. They are recruited from the staff of Neapolitan schools and are individually selected on the basis of their previous experience and degree of motivation. They come from various tiers of the educational system—the primary, middle, and secondary levels. This special composition, designed to cover the lacunae in the children's basic learning skills, has also proved to be important in psychological terms.

The project also has a sizeable team of psychologists who provide teachers and the other professionals involved with support in acquiring relational skills adequate to contain the anxieties stemming from contact with such difficult children. Providing a theoretical framework and a network of relationships between the various institutions and professions involved is a central task.

We thought that the students needed "a maturational environment", not individual treatment, since their limited capacities for acknowledging and verbalizing their feelings would impede their benefiting from counselling or psychotherapy. Moreover, given the high percentage of mothers who suffer from mental health problems and are receiving pharmacological treatment, we thought that any offer of treatment might be perceived by the students as confirmation not only that they were backward from the academic point of view, but that, more generally, something was wrong with their minds. We have tried to help the teachers to expand the therapeutic function of their role, by creating spaces specifically devoted to helping the young people to express and reflect on their feelings, such as "circle time" and "special time".

The concept of containment in the educational relationship

Shirley Hoxter's paper "The Old Woman Who Lived in a Shoe" (1981) explored the explosive effect that deprived young people's needs and mental states can have on teachers and school structure. She used the image of the shoe, borrowed from a children's nursery rhyme, as a metaphor for a collapsed container whose bonds and structure are inadequate and in a state of disrepair. Teachers and students—the old woman and her children—live in a state of reciprocal persecution in which psychic pain, which cannot be contained and healed, is mutually inflicted and becomes increasingly magnified.

Hoxter applied the Bionian concept of containment (1962a) to the analysis of the relationship between schools and students; in particular, she focused on Bion's description of the three types of link between the container and the contained (1970). In the link termed "symbiotic", the container and contained correspond to each other and modify each other, to their reciprocal advantage. In the "commensal" link, container and contained coexist, but neither of the two has a significant effect on the other. In the "parasitic" link, the relationship between container and contained proves to be destructive for both members of the pair.

> One can consider what must be contained, the living children, with their emotions, their needs, the pure strength of their drive towards development, as an explosive force, to which educational and social systems provide the coercive frameworks in the form of schools and other institutions. In some schools, which are seemingly well ordered and which I will refer to as conventional

> schools, control of the explosive force of children's emotions may be obtained, to quote Bion, "by making use of such boring forms of expression that they will fail to express any kind of meaning." Nevertheless it is extremely likely that in such a school there is very little space for the sort of child who cannot adapt, whose mere presence represents a challenge, the child who has physical and mental needs, defects or qualities that are too pressing to be obliterated in the prevailing absence of meaning. Consequently such a child tends to be expelled from conventional schools to special units. [Bion, 1970, p. 5]

Hoxter's analysis demonstrates that there is no "good-enough" school in itself, no more than there exists a "good-enough" mother, independent of the specific characteristics of the child. Limited maternal capacities can blossom in the presence of an easy, facilitating child, while a child with problems or with a high level of intolerance of frustration can easily exhaust the resources of an "average" mother. The opposite is also true, so that reduced maternal capacities can lead to the failure of the relationship with an "average" child, while a mother who has unusual containment capacities can cope with the impact of an extremely difficult child and support the maximum potential development of the child.

The reference to the concept of containment and its implications has, from the very outset, represented a founding element of our approach, focusing attention on the quality of the relationships between individuals and systems that are, reciprocally, container and contained and on the factors that are capable of strengthening or undermining the structure of containment at macro- and micro-levels.

The composition of the psychotherapy team

When we were asked to join the Project, concerning ourselves with the training of the teachers and what would soon be termed the "maintenance of the human and professional resources", it was made clear to us that the nature of the task required a team that had a range of experience but also a fundamental coherence. Our conviction that this was right was strengthened by a powerful image that came into our minds during one of our first meetings. It concerned images of a film, "The Dirty Dozen", in which a band of desperadoes is recruited for an extremely risky mission. The training of the band takes place through the obsessively repeated learning of rigidly articulated tasks so that they can be carried out automatically. The story ends with the task completed but at the cost of the death of most of the band! In the film, the learning imparted to the individuals who must act as a cohesive unit takes place through a form of training that leaves no space for thought or individual creativity. This has the advantage of being efficient in terms of time but leaves many dead on the battlefield. A different metaphor, with respect to the composition of a group faced with an exceptional effort, comes from the autobiography of Peter Brook. In this case, the source was one of Grimm's fairy tales.

> The young hero must save the princess but his resources are not sufficient; he needs special qualities which only others possess. He therefore forms a group. One of them can see an ant at an incredible distance, another member can hear the sound of a pin dropping from many miles away, while a third can drink the entire contents of a lake; another member can feel warmth when it is cold and cold when it is warm. They eventually form a group of seven men who undertake a mission that no one man could achieve on his own" [Brook, 1998, p. 157]

This metaphor conveyed to us the main qualities that had to be put together in the group and in each individual. In work with highly deprived children, Winnicott (1984) emphasizes the importance of the psychologist being able to "survive": "Your job is to survive. In this setting the word 'survive' means not only that you live through it and that you manage not to get damaged, but also that you are not provoked into vindictiveness". Survival, therefore, refers to the need to safeguard one's own psychic structure and capacity for containment, and to be able to think and be helpful even in difficult situations. The capacity to "feel warmth when it is cold and cool when it is warm" powerfully evokes the need to maintain an appropriate "emotional temperature", infusing warmth in dead and stale relationships or cooling hot emotions. This implies coping with sudden and unexpected swings in mood, as often happens with deprived children.

Similarly, the capacity of another member to "drink the entire contents of a lake" suggests the need to provide space for experiences and suffering that go beyond ordinary human capacities. Grimm's fairy tale refers to sharpened qualities of observation that extend our capacity to see and hear "facts" that cannot immediately be perceived by the senses. Observations from a psychoanalytic standpoint can, indeed, transform "observed facts into meaningful thoughts capable of producing growth in meaning" (Oliva, 1987).

A model of concentric containers

Our model is represented by a set of concentric settings designed to contain the relationships between the various individuals, groups, and agencies involved. Apart from the work discussion seminars, which will be described later in some detail, these involved the following:

a The inter-professional and inter-institutional Co-ordinating Group, which meets fortnightly for two hours; its main aim is to hold the project together through recognizing the internal and external forces that tend to split and fragment it. The attempt to preserve a reflective perspective even in the heat of conflict through openly recognizing and addressing conflicts represents a new and unusual way of handling institutional and professional relationships that are generally merely acted out and/or bureaucratized.

b Theory Seminars take place four times a year. They represent an opportunity to share and conceptualize experience and to listen to multidisciplinary theoretical contributions. These seminars help the educational staff to feel part of a wider community that can reflect on the issues with which they are confronted in their daily work and enrich and strengthen their understanding of them. This is crucial for reinforcing the teachers' identity, which can be shaken both by the students' contempt and negativity and by the loss of more traditional professional approaches and points of reference.

c A Discussion Group open to everyone takes place at the end of the Theory Seminars. It aims to highlight group phenomena triggered by the work with teenage drop-outs. It provides an opportunity to gain experience in the "here and now" of the group dynamics activated in the groups involved in the Project.

d A Supervision Group for the psychological team had not been envisaged in the original project, but it was soon introduced to meet the need felt by the psychotherapists to have such a space. In many ways the Chance Project represented a new experience: we were not offering consultancy to an institution in crisis, but contributing to the development of an atypical institution embodying educational and therapeutic aspects.

The place of work discussion seminars

A Swiss educationalist, Mireille Cifali, writes in her book entitled *Le lien éducatif: Contre-jour psychanalytique*:

> The more an (educational) institution addresses the question of suffering on a daily basis, the more anxiety tends to increase and the sense of impotence takes root, the greater is the benefit that can derive from creating spaces for thinking, symbolising and sublimating. If it does not prove possible to find a "place" for metabolising suffering and anxiety, these remain individual experiences which are lost to transforming reflection and discussion" (p. 152). This "place for negotiating conflicts" and for "letting words circulate" also becomes a place where it is possible to "deconstruct received ideas, ready-made sentences and deceptively attractive commonplaces, and search for original reflections from beyond the well-trodden paths. [Cifali, 1994, p. 100]

We could not find more appropriate words to describe the need that initially drove us to think about how all the staff involved in the daily work could meet on a regular basis. As Cifali observes, teachers tend to ask for "explanations" of the behaviour of young people from which to derive indications about the right response. Replacing explanation with understanding means placing oneself in the subjective field.

> The act of understanding engages thought in the dimension of intersubjectivity. [It is necessary] to talk about what has happened, detach oneself from the situation, describe it . . . and share the experience without being afraid. [One needs to] abdicate from omnipotence, let slip the mask of a supposedly ideal situation, and observe, describe, avoid remaining on the outside, grasp what little there is to understand, and accept the part that remains incomprehensible. The clinical approach defines the outlines of a space in which practice discovers the possibility of theorization, beginning from a specific situation. [Cifali, 1994, p. 286]

Facing the task

We organized a work discussion seminar within the three schools, each convened by a child psychotherapist. The seminars take place on a fortnightly basis simultaneously at each school, to allow the possibility of shared activities on those Wednesdays when there are no seminars. They were intended to enable the discussion of work situations described in turn by the participants, focusing in particular on the teacher–adolescent relationship. In emphasizing observation, there was a distinct awareness that, rather than the impartial and distant eye of an expert, these young people needed an affectionate and steady adult gaze that did not flinch when faced with emptiness or desperate violence, and which did not send back signals of failures in understanding. Such a benevolent gaze might grasp sparks of life, hidden potential, fragments of skills on which to build when faced with life catastrophes ostentatiously displayed or ill-concealed by silence (Adamo et al., 2005).

Mobilizing observation has, however, taken place gradually and with difficulty. For a long time the seminar leaders were confronted with an absence of observation and the need to try to understand the complex underlying dynamics. In this regard, one might suggest a parallel with psychotherapeutic work carried out with severely disturbed children who do not use a symbolic dimension in their communication and therefore require the therapist to employ a different technique from that used with children who are able to play or who display neurotic inhibitions. In leading work discussion seminars, one has to be prepared to cope with the anxieties evoked by the observation and discussion of one's work with others, but it was disorienting when the proposed task turned out to be invested with such powerful anxieties that it was actively attacked or abandoned. This provided a mirror image of what took place on the "battlefield" between the teachers and the young people.

Grasping what had happened to the teachers, who had had to learn how to cope with the students' rejection of structured teaching activities, it proved crucial for the seminar leaders to avoid entrenching themselves behind a sterile defence of the task. The Chance teachers were encountering feelings of impotence, inadequacy, anger, fear, discouragement, and uncertainty. What they felt was at stake, and under attack was their deepest sense of personal and professional identity. This stirred up profound primitive anxieties. At the beginning of the work, talking about this raised a storm of protest. There is a widespread tendency among teachers to deny anxiety, which "is viewed as a sign of weakness which would betray their incompetence" (Cifali, 1994, p. 94). Yet "the profession exposes one to anxiety". In Chance these anxieties were intensified by the sense of challenge that the project represented, by the fact that the professionals had been chosen on the basis of their experience and skills, by the fear of failure, and by the excessive workload deriving from omnipotent expectations and persecutory feelings of guilt.

A further source of difficulty was linked to the fact that observational methodology is largely extraneous to the practice and culture of the traditional school. The habit of working behind closed doors in the classroom and the evaluative aspect of the teacher's function contribute to making teachers particularly vulnerable to others' gaze, which is dreaded as intrusive and judgemental.

In the early stages the teachers often described how young people tore up photos taken of their productions and destroyed their work. The gaze of others evokes the fear of a gaze felt to be critical and spoiling, a selective gaze that takes in and conveys only the image of one's failings. A scene from a documentary film made about the Chance project, entitled "*Pesci combattenti*" [Fighting Fishes], illustrates this. Faced with the eye of the video camera filming a scene, a teenage boy complained: "Get rid of this bloody video camera, you're just making me look like a complete cretin." This expectation was certainly linked to negative and belittling experiences encountered in previous schools and reinforced by the cultural background, where looking at someone is considered an insult, a form of violence, which can provoke aggressive verbal or physical response.

In talking so insistently about teenagers who felt violated by the gaze of others, the teachers were also alluding to their own vulnerability. The similarity of feeling among students and teachers interfered with containment, since the persecutory anxieties remained unmodified or were intensified in daily interaction. Once, when we distributed an account of a classroom observation as an example of the type of observations that they might make, some of them expressed violent indignation at what they felt to be the university's intention to conduct research by exploiting their work.

Another possible consequence of the splitting and projection of reflective capacities is an imitative identification with the "expert" and a tendency to talk about one's own experience through the language of others or in jargon. However, the most painful and disturbing aspects of the teachers' experience tended to be reproduced in the group, and this could be explored in the relationship with the seminar leader. Diffident silence or limited and formal exchange conveyed the dilemma and impotence teachers felt when faced with students who seemed to lack even a minimal sense of curiosity or interest in learning. The dynamics behind the students' daily attacks, dismissiveness, provocation, confusion, and excitement were reproduced in the seminars. Noise and confusion, the use of bad language and jokes with sexual overtones, created a rowdy and chaotic atmosphere. This made it extremely difficult to think and maintain an internal equilibrium based on receptivity and reverie; instead, it drove one to react, since the situation was not represented but reproduced. To describe this situation, Freud (1915a) once used the metaphor of a play where, instead of watching the scene of a fire on stage, one finds oneself involved in a real fire raging in the theatre. In the seminars, the teachers brought their experience with the students and re-enacted the students' transference towards them of incompetent, impotent, abusive, or abused figures.

Sometimes, even just a window looking onto the street when left open produced a sort of disturbing sensorial bombardment:

> Wednesday afternoon, meeting of the Work Discussion Seminar: the chaotic and deafening noises of the street enter the room imperiously and threaten any possibility of communication. The music of the local Neapolitan pop songs merges with the calls of street-sellers and mothers, with the smells of meat sauce and freshly washed sheets. Everything in the room seems to merge and get confused and it is impossible to protect oneself from this chaotic noise, to sort out what is happening in the group: this clearly echoes what happens in the morning in Chance classes. [Adamo Serpieri, Giusti, Portanova, & Tamajo, 2003, p. 67]

The sensorial bombardment, absence of boundaries, and inextricable confusion powerfully entered the seminar space and the minds of the leaders. The teachers' request, occasionally put forward quite consciously, was to share their suffering "You come here once in a while and expect to understand. . . . You must suffer with us." The qualities of the container that have proved to be especially necessary, given the nature of the work, are many. Continuity, resilience, the capacity to receive and cope with violent and abusive language and behaviour, with attacks aimed at making one feel impotent and deskilled, with sexual excitement, provocativeness, intrusiveness, and violation of boundaries, extreme emotional temperatures and sudden variations of it, flexibility, tolerance, creativity, and hopefulness are some of these.

A story with several voices

In the initial phase of work, the seminar leaders' reverie was mainly aimed at grasping small signs of creative thinking. This is analogous to what takes place in the development of language, where the mother bestows meaning on the baby's pre-speech, enabling access to the spoken word. Paraphrasing Bion, we could say that what was produced in the group frequently bore resemblance to "doodles in sound" (Bion, 1963, p. 52). Gradually, fuller accounts began to make their appearance and were enriched, during the discussion, by collective contributions. It seemed that the capacity to think about disturbing emotions was made possible by the concrete presence of the seminar leader, as in early childhood, when the possibility of the child starting to think instead of evacuating disturbing emotional experiences requires the physical presence of the mother. Shared narration enabled the seminar to function as a cradle of the capacity to notice, gradually enabling the sequence of events to be reconstructed and emotions to be expressed and reflected on. In this way, it proved possible to move from outpourings and the search for magical and immediate solutions towards thinking together.

Often we began with an urgent discussion about how to cope with an immediate emergency; gradually it became possible to create more space and to gather pieces of understanding that could guide teachers' responses. Staff began to store up experience and develop forms of shared work, which laid the foundation for good practice. When this happened and could be made explicit, the sense of relief was evident. By way of illustration, we present the following situation, which was described verbally by the participants:

> During the meeting a particularly difficult recent day is discussed. Three boys and two girls had barricaded themselves into the staff room two days previously after a ceremony in which flowers were given to the staff for "Women's day", giving no hint as to what would happen later. The staff tried several times to persuade the students to relent but found themselves up against an increasingly deaf and unswerving opposition. It was decided to summon the parents so that they could collect their children. When they heard this, the students left the room in which they were barricaded, accused the teachers of betrayal, and became even more destructive and uncontainable: desks and cupboards were overturned, and foul language was directed against the staff. After a while, it seemed that the worst was over. However, this proved to be an illusion, because the insistent stares of staff from the host school—who were witnesses to the events—were regarded by the students as intrusive and tantamount to provocation. The atmosphere became even more uncontainable, and pupils began

> hurling insults and seeking a physical clash with these outsiders. With great difficulty, the Chance staff managed to prevent the event from degenerating still further; the students were persuaded to return and have lunch. The day concluded without further incident.
>
> In discussion it was not possible at first to move away from a heated debate about how to re-establish the rules that had to be observed. The seminar leader asked the staff about their own feelings. One teacher expressed pain at the behaviour of the students just when they had seemed to be reaping the first rewards of their shared efforts. Another expressed disappointment and guilt at resorting to parental intervention, feeling that this had contributed to exacerbating the clash. The staff seemed to oscillate between two positions—the stance of a parent who, after expending enormous energy, sees his or her expectations dashed at the realization that the child is not what he or she had wanted, and a profound tendency to devalue themselves and their role, having overestimated themselves and underestimated the difficulties facing them. Others expressed a sense of failure, tiredness, and loss of motivation and the need for more help. This led the seminar leader to describe two points of view: on the one hand, their pain led to the desire to understand and to examine the causes of events; on the other, there was a prevailing sense that a rupture had taken place, and they no longer felt able to cope or had the energy to carry on. She emphasized the importance of linking these events to the students' adolescent preoccupations, both libidinal and aggressive. It emerged that this is particularly difficult with students such as those in the Chance Project, who constantly search for a limit and, at the same time, are not in the least prepared to respect it. Finding oneself in such a situation represents a very difficult test and proves a gruelling experience.

Here were the first tentative attempts at reconstructing the event in a temporal sequence, identifying turning points, and recognizing the many different feelings and positions of the staff. Not yet clear is how an affectionate exchange—the giving of flowers to the teachers—could turn into the start of a revolt. Yet this is a recurrent aspect of work with deprived children (Boston & Szur, 1969), an expression of their fear at having their rejecting and disdainful defensive armour dented and at discovering their vulnerability in a dependent relationship, with all the associated risk of further disappointment.

Writing things down

Participants gradually became aware of the possibility of bringing in their own feelings, without feeling excessively threatened. They began to produce observations that reconstructed a small sequence or condensed a problematic episode, where they were personally involved.

An example is provided by the following material, which deals with an episode involving Luca, a youth tutor who belongs to a religious community.

> Luca describes how everything began from a series of verbal attacks made by Ciro, who usually behaves more calmly. Immediately afterwards Nello tried to attack Luca physically and to pull down his trousers. Luca wanted to discuss what had happened with the students in order to prevent them thinking that he had made accusations against them that led to the three-day suspension imposed. After listening to the various comments, the seminar leader observes that this was not the first time that episodes of this kind had taken place: she therefore asks whether Luca might serve as a magnet for students' feelings and anxieties. In the gesture of pulling down the trousers, done as a sort of joke, the students may be conveying their difficulty in understanding Luca's choice of calling, and thus offloading their anxieties about sexuality onto him. One of the teachers observes that Luca tends to place too much emphasis on the students' behaviour. Another highlights the problem for the youth tutors who act as go-betweens, an interface between teachers and students. The seminar leader comments that this meeting is pervaded by an atmosphere of kindness and honesty, which makes it possible to comprehend Luca's difficulty and to reflect together on possible meanings of the event without confining themselves to matters of discipline.

Observations like this gave the sense of growth at both an individual and a group level; they represented an act of individual responsibility and trust in the group, each individual feeling he or she could bring their own contribution.

Gradually, written observations were produced, such as the following example taken from a science lesson, revealing teacher fallibility:

> Enzo is fascinated by volcanoes, and he touches the stones. I ask him if he recognizes any of them. He picks one up and says, "It's

> an ordinary stone." I tell him that it's a pumice stone; you can tell because it's so light. I point out to him the difference in weight compared to the fossil and observe that pumice stones sometimes float on the sea. Enzo refuses to believe this. We decide to do an experiment to see if it floats. We fill a glass tank with water and ask Enzo to place the stone in the water: the stone sinks to the bottom. Enzo looks at me with a satisfied expression; I am nonplussed. My grandmother, the former owner of the stone, had told me 40 years ago that it was a pumice stone, and I had never checked to see if it was true! I congratulate Enzo on his intuition and thank him for making me test my hypothesis and draw a conclusion. [Magliulo, 2003, p. 124]

Self-observation

Infant and young child observation demonstrate that the presence of an observer can help to develop the observational capacities of mother and child. In our experience, a similar process may not only take place in individual teachers, but extend to an entire institution and come to form part of its culture and pedagogical practice. The building of this shared culture draws on several aspects of our methodology. For example, in the fortnightly educational meetings, concern for the maintenance of a constant setting became evident, and elements began to appear in the teachers' accounts that could be defined as meta-observations, signalling a process of gradual introjection. A youth tutor, for instance, introduces his observation with the following consideration:

> "I had so many tangled thoughts in my head, and I am still very confused, disappointed, and angry about what happened. I just hope that talking about it here with you serves some purpose; however, I've noticed that the mere fact of writing it out beforehand helped me feel a bit better."

The act of thinking and writing here acquires an important meaning, since what are initially defined as "tangled thoughts" are transformed into named and differentiated emotions: confusion, disappointment, anger. The beneficial effect of this process is felt and recognized by the tutor himself.

The importance of sharing thoughts with other staff within the seminar is shown by the following comment of a "social mother":

"I took part in my first psychology meeting in the Chance project without really appreciating what its aim was. During my first period spent in Chance, I had accumulated so many doubts, anxieties, and fears that I was not able to cope with the numerous situations of tension and attacks from the students. During the meetings with the psychologist, teachers and other members of staff expressed their emotions through the reconstruction of events, and I felt heartened: we all shared the same problems."

This excerpt from a dialogue between two art teachers demonstrates more sophisticated thinking:

> These children have a stereotyped idea of beauty; if we can compare their eyes to the camera lens, it is as though the focus had remained stuck on a particular image: this image appears when they are given another image—and it is this image, and this one alone, which they draw on the sheet of paper.
>
> When we go outside and take photographs, holding their hands, suggesting what to observe, talking together, is like applying a drop of oil to a blocked lens, it suddenly begins to collect fresh images.
>
> At that point you can even show them Chagall or Picasso or Mirò: knowing that great artists, about whom they had no prior knowledge, used "strange" colours, out-of-proportion images, and dared to express their dreams, enables the child, who may have many dreams but is unable to express them, to look at his or her work with conviction, with bright eyes and the smile of one who is satisfied with him/herself: you see those shining eyes. . . . [Adamo, Iannazzone, Melazzini, & Peyron, 2005, pp. 97–98]

The "block" refers to the defensive mechanisms that act as a constraint upon the vision of others, of oneself, of the world, flattening it and restricting it; however, the "lubrication" provided by a cautious but ongoing provision of new emotional experience can widen the cognitive and emotional horizon.

The methodology of observation has also acquired an important role in the selection of students. A project designed to accept young people who have been excluded from school has an intrinsic difficulty in selection, which can so easily be felt as a further type of exclusion. It stirs guilt because Chance is often the last hope these adolescents have before ending up in a community home. The experience accumulated over the years has made the staff aware of the risk of omnipotence that frequently lurks behind difficulties in selection. An important measure eventually introduced was the inclusion of a third staff member in the admission interviews with the young people, which are conducted by a teacher–youth tutor pair; this person acts as a non-participant observer. Their reports represent an important contribution to the decision-making process. For example, the trembling hand of a teenager, who may seem cocky and aggressive, highlights his fear and fragility, while pauses or changes in topic may indicate conflictual areas that it would be useful to investigate further (Adamo & Aiello, 2006).

Ups and downs

We are aware of the risk of giving a false impression of Chance as an ideal context in which the working-through of emotions and conflicts in a stable way is established. Nothing could be further from the truth. A recent crisis will serve as comparison with the earlier episode of "insurrection and barricading".

A boy named Luigi failed to turn up for school after the Christmas holidays; on the following day news arrived of the death of his father at the hands of a *Camorra* punitive mission.

The following account is taken from a teacher's observation.

> The school is almost empty and would remain this way the whole week; no more than seven or eight students came in each day. During the Wednesday assembly, one of us made an attempt to comment on the events and stated that sometimes innocent people get killed. The students' response was drastic: "If someone is killed, they've done something serious"; "The *Camorra*", says Giuseppe, "always gives you another chance." The students say they are convinced that Luigi will never return to school. Some ask to go the funeral to show their comradeship with their classmate. We manage to say that it is a tragic and delicate fact that . . . the funeral will be "policed". A long silence follows. Rosa's eyes blaze, and she proposes writing to Luigi.
>
> Luigi's closest school friends did not take part in the assembly and later refuse to enter the room to discuss the matter with the tutor, remaining outside. One of them describes what happened with a certain air of detachment, as though he were reading a newspaper; another recounts episodes of exemplary punishment that "had to be done" because: "Miss, people are making more mistakes

> (meaning that they disobey the *Camorra*'s rules) all the time", but immediately afterwards he adds: "If they did that to my Dad, I'd get out the Kalashnikov."

These are excerpts from the seminar following the incident. The main view of the staff was their painful certainty that the boy would never return to school, an emblematic experience of a feeling of failure and catastrophe. Faced with the evidence of *Camorra* involvement of many of the students' relatives, either as victims or as executioners, the fear was expressed that the "safe haven represented up till that point by Chance might become a theatre of war", and that this might provoke contagious abandonment of school. However, the staff tried to encourage the students to work through what had happened; they attempted to talk about the young people's responses, even those that were most disturbing for them, such as the declarations of their identification with the *Camorra*.

The seminar began talking about how one of the most uncontainable youths, Carmine, spoke about his wish to die.

> His words came out in a whisper, while he was copying the figure of a dragon, to which he added an enormous tongue of flame coming out of its mouth. He adds that he doesn't want to go home but to sleep in the park. Lello says that he slept the night there in the summer. Maria remarks that you can see the cemetery from the park. Lello lies down on the table and assumes the position of a corpse.

Luigi did return to school, initially welcomed with great anxiety by the other students, almost as if he were the bearer of a dangerous infection.

> During the assembly following his return, there is a lot of unrest. A girl runs outside and asks for her tutor: she tells her of her anxiety about her father: "I'm afraid that my father will end up the same way when he comes out of prison: they're waiting for him." Two of the social mothers recount how some of the students deserted assembly and, in the main hall, enacted the killing of a person who had betrayed the clan: "Three boys sat down, one behind the other, on two chairs; they pretended to sniff drugs, then they started driving their 'motorbike'; their expressions and body language were full of ruthless violence as they drove fast, making

> the roar of the engine with their voices. They reached their target, played by a fourth student, called him a traitor, and, holding a door-handle with the pin sticking out in front like a pistol, cried: 'You bastard, you've made a mistake and you're going to die', and 'shot' him."

From then on and for many months these themes returned repeatedly and reminded us of the working-through of a traumatic bereavement. The teachers described moments when the students, while talking calmly in an intimate context such as the tutorial group, recalled experiences, such as the loss of a baby brother, a mother's abortions, or the painful operations that followed a childhood illness.

After several meetings that focused on more general questions, Patrizia today reads an observation entitled "Handles and pins" .

> This refers to a new student "game", which consists in wrenching off door handles and using them as pistols. The observation contains an extremely vivid description of the way each of the students involved perceives the handles. During the discussion, a teacher says that the students are still enacting the death of Luigi's father, while another says that although it is a pretty tasteless game, it is one that the students feel they can bring to Chance because it is contained and tolerated.
>
> It emerges in discussion that the students' interest in door handles goes back many months; they had long used them to shut themselves in or shut others in or out, but they also tended to appropriate them and hide them. This also happens with other objects in the school, in particular cakes and snacks. Hiding things is usually a prelude to their disappearance.
>
> It is therefore a "game" that seems to be connected to the question of power: about who decides when to open and shut doors, about how much good food there is—themes that represent the daily life of Chance. It is now clear that since the death of Luigi's father the game has become more violent.
>
> The social mothers report that in this period the hunt for the handles, which the students refer to as *"ferro"* (literally "iron", but used to refer to pistols in *Camorra* jargon) increasingly takes on the semblance of a quest for power, that of the *Camorra* boss. Other comments show how violent episodes are escalating and how chaos frequently seems to reign. During the discussion, it

> emerges that this makes the staff feel threatened, overwhelmed, and provoked, and that this has made it difficult to realize that the handle game had actually taken on the dimension of destructive gang behaviour (Williams, 1990). The gang rebels against the rules of Chance, perceived at that moment as both rich and mean, thus stimulating greed and anger and the need to attack.

We believe that this description, based on several meetings of the group, reveals the capacity of the staff to avoid "turning a blind eye" (Steiner, 1982) to external family involvement and to the even more disturbing internal identifications of the young people with the system and logic of the *Camorra*. Nevertheless, their capacity to "survive"—that is, their capacity to preserve their emotional availability without retreating—enables the students to make contact with and express sadder feelings. Observation also makes it possible to grasp the reverberations of these events in the dynamics of the peer group and to comprehend how the symbolic framework of the game deteriorates under the impact of the anxieties about the long summer holiday in prospect.

Conclusions

During a meeting of the Coordinating group, a member of staff described an event that had taken place some time ago. The Chance project had been chosen by the Council of Europe as one of the six best European projects designed to combat school truancy. The presentation of the final research report (Hardiman & Lapeyre, 2004; Lapeyre, 2004) was to be made at Strasbourg, and a representative group of teachers and pupils had been invited to take part. It was the first time that the Chance project students had travelled in a plane, and they were excited and anxious. The teachers were seated so that each of them was sitting next to a student. During the flight, one of the students, who until that moment had been absorbed in contemplating the sky from the window, turned to the teacher and, with a sense of surprise, said that he had never imagined that when it was not sunny, if one changed position, as was happening to them now flying at high altitude, the clouds remained below, and the sun began to shine once more. The teacher was struck by the boy's comment, and it struck us all. It seemed to us to convey the essence of our work: to bring light into the students' lives, widen their horizons, give them a glimpse of other possible perspectives, distance them from the darkness that looms over their lives, offer them the experience of a stable environment and of caring adults, which could be borne in mind even in the dark moments that their lives would continue to hold in store. The boy's words exemplify a mutually enriching relationship between words and emotions, adult and child, young people and the Project. It is a symbiotic relationship of containment.

The meaning of our work can be summarized like this: the creation of an experimental school, which accepts young people who have been prematurely scarred, in which students and all the staff involved can be offered opportunities to have authentic encounters with themselves and others, a place where words and silence can become true forms of communication, and in which it is possible to accept darkness and light in others, within oneself, within one's own history and in the surrounding reality.

Note

We wish to thank warmly the colleagues who have in the past years shared this work with us, enriching our thinking with their contributions: they are Professor Paolo Valerio, co-planner of the Psychological Project and co-responsible for it in the years 1998–2005; Professor Guelfo Margherita, leader of the discussion group and supervisor of the psychological team; and Dr Flavia Portanova, seminar leader in one of the work discussion seminars.

Our deepest thanks also go to all the teachers, educators, and other professionals of the Chance Project for allowing us to share in this difficult and inspirational experience.

CHAPTER TEN

Work discussion seminars with the staff of a children's home for street children in Puebla, Mexico

Gianna Williams

This chapter describes the use of work discussion in Casa Juconi, a home for street children in Mexico that I have visited and kept in touch with regularly over the past eight years.

Juconi stands for "*junto con los niños*" [together with the children], and Juconi is an NGO devoted to "retrieving" street children and bringing them to Casa Juconi—a very unusual children's home—for a long stay. Casa Juconi is unusual because it has opened itself to a keen interest in the *emotional* life of the street children, and this is *not* a frequent occurrence in the many organizations devoted to street children's welfare in Latin America. I have been to Puebla, the town where Casa Juconi is located, six times for an average period of ten days, since 1999. My work with the group started with my presence in Puebla—but it has continued with "distance teaching", via email, during the intervals between visits. I have been joined in the task of "distance teaching" by two child psychotherapy colleagues. There are regular staff meetings where our email input is discussed by the group.

I focus here on just one particular aspect of my work: talking with the educators, the teachers, the house parents—in fact, all the people involved in the care and education of the children, as well as those maintaining contact with external agencies and with the children's natural parents when that was possible. We discussed two children every day, one for three and half hours in the morning and one for three and half hours in the afternoon. All those present in the room and acquainted with the child in question took part in talking about him (I say about "him" because there are only boys, 24 of them, between the ages of 7 and 18, in Casa Juconi).

In 1999 I introduced for the first time the idea of "Special Times" with the individual children. These consisted in weekly encounters that took place in the same place at the same time for 45 minutes. Each child has a "Special Time" box with drawing materials, and so on. Whatever the child writes or draws in the session is kept in his "Special Time" box.

My experience of work discussion seminars on "Special Times" carried out in very different contexts dates from 1975, when I took my first work discussion seminar in what is now the Tavistock Course in Psychoanalytic Observational Studies.

The Special Times in Juconi House had to be adapted to the resources available. Those are as yet limited and therefore also limited is the amount of time the children have for Special Time, which is now a standard period of one year. We came to realize that people involved in the Special Time should not be those directly involved in the daily care of the children. The educators are asked to listen, to give their full attention to the child, not to set an agenda for the session, not to ask many questions, just to see what the child is prepared to bring. Some children are silent for a long time and very difficult to reach, much like the "doubly deprived" children I wrote about a long time ago (Henry, 1974). Other children are very responsive to the offer of help. One can formulate the hypothesis that, however gloomy their history, these children may have had some good days at the beginning of their lives. Most of the children are Indios, and Indio mothers carry their children on their backs in such a way that they can turn and see their face and thus have eye as well as body contact with them. Pedro, the child I am going to describe, might well have had one of these good starts in life.

We discussed Pedro, an 11-year-old child, when I last went to Puebla in December 2006. He had already been in Casa Juconi for one year when I visited. One knew with certainty that he had been physically abused by his father and that both his parents were addicted to alcohol. He was the third of four children, and they had all been severely neglected. We do not know for how long he had lived on the street before he agreed to come into Casa Juconi. (The befriending of street children by educators can take many months; the children are aware of many dangers, including the one of organ traffic.) Pedro had certainly attended school and could read and write. Although his parents have been contacted, there is very little likelihood that Pedro will return home.

Pedro is not an unreachable child. He responded to the offer of "Special Time" in a wholehearted way and told his educator a great deal about himself. This was in the shape of stories that he dictated during his "Special Time" sessions. The stories suggested a great deal about the internal world and, possibly, the history of this child. They developed gradually and initially showed strong defences against the risk of softness.

I will give an example from one of the early stories. The main character is called Sylvester.

> Pedro says about Sylvester: "Sylvester does not like hugs. Sylvester must be frightened of being hugged. He runs away when someone tries to cuddle him. He runs away and gets very tired and very thirsty."

At this point in the story, when he is tired and thirsty, Sylvester becomes softer: we see him running to a place called "*Abuelita*" [little grandmother]. This is the name Pedro gives to the children's home and to all working in it and for it. It is interesting that "Abuelita" is a collective name, certainly not openly referring just to the house mother, Bibiana.

Sylvester, the child who does not want to be cuddled, fears the danger of too close a relationship. He can only relate to the impersonal object "Abuelita" when he is thirsty and he needs his thirst to be quenched and thus feels a little softer.

Pedro was able to give the educator a very poignant description of the predicament of the children in the children's home. Again quoting from one of his stories:

> "Those children have no mother, they have only little grandmother. When one of them gets hurt, he is looked after by little grandmother, and all the children in this children's home are very hurt and need a lot of looking after."

We are perhaps getting closer to "Abuelita" having something to do with the house mother, Bibiana, but the "Special Time" person, a very sensitive woman, Sandra Cortes, was able to respect Pedro's defences and did not make a direct link with the house mother, even when it became quite obvious. Pedro was probably involved in gang dynamics when he was a street child. The gang does not agree with any of its members being softies and being aware of needing looking after.

The gang members in the street would probably laugh at Pedro if they saw him getting too close to the housemother.

In one of the stories, the gang, which at this point I think represents an internal gang, returns to claim Pedro's membership. With the gang, Pedro goes to a place on top of the world—*"arriba del mundo"*. Pedro, as the main character of the stories, at this point called Marvin, at times visits his "friends" (gang members) because, he says, *"they are street children like him"*, but one can see that he is no longer really a street child. I will quote from the story:

> "Marvin likes to go on top of the world, because on top of the world he has friends who are just like him, but Marvin lived with Abuelita and he only *visited* his friends. He did not like to live with them, because he did not like it very much there. In this place it is terribly cold, because the place that is on top of the world is very cold. The friends of Marvin's could live there because they had a space ship (*a gang hideout?*)."

It is very important that Abuelita worries about Pedro being drawn back into the hideout of the gang (so many children feel tempted to go back to the street), and it is very important for the educators to be aware of this danger.

> "Abuelita thinks at times that Marvin could remain up there and asks the others: where is Marvin? Marvin comes back to Abuelita and tells her that he has come back, and he will not remain up there. He will always return to Abuelita."

So we learn that he is even thinking about Abuelita when he is on top of the world.

> "Marvin flew up and arrived on top of the world. He went as high as one of the stars and brought it down. He was going to give this star to Abuelita, because Abuelita loved stars. Abuelita looked at the star and thanked him. Then he went out to play."

He feels a family child again.

This part of the story tells us something about Pedro's relationship with Abuelita (and possibly also of his experience as a baby), which is evocative of an experience of "aesthetic reciprocity" (Meltzer, 1988) between infant and mother. In a state of "aesthetic reciprocity" an infant might well feel that his mother's eyes are like stars.

Abuelita is now getting dangerously close to being equated with the house mother. For instance, Abuelita is described as playing ball games and assigning tasks to the children on Monday—all aspects of the house mother that make her extremely recognizable. Still she must be called Abuelita.

The children's home is very different from a gang hideout. In one of the stories we hear a description that gives evidence of the children feeling membership of a group rather than a gang (Williams, 1997), a group where painful feelings can be shared.

> "Those good friends play hide and seek and football, and they talk about what they feel. They help one another, asking each other: 'How are things? Can I give you a hand?' They also talk about their families and about something sad, like the fact that their mothers are not coming to visit them. They are sad, and so they talk with a friend. The friend tells them, 'Let's go and play. One of these days your family will come to visit you.'"

In the story the main character has not seen his family for *two weeks*. At this point Pedro had not seen his family for months.

We see one of Pedro's defences returning when we hear about a little animal who would like to lose its head because it gives the little animal a lot of worries. Is there a wish in Pedro to stop thinking?—thinking about where and why it hurts, as it did when he spoke about his mother not visiting? The wish to lose one's head suggests an attack on linking, but Pedro is not *devoted* to "attacks on linking" (Bion, 1967). He is just protecting himself occasionally from very painful feelings; at other times he faces his feelings filtered through the symbolic function of his narratives.

The sunny picture of the children's group in the children's home does not tell us the whole story about Pedro's feelings. The real story is that he would like to be an only child. Sharing with others evokes a host of difficult feelings. In one of the stories Coyote is an only child. Coyote goes to look for Abuelita at the market and does not find her. He comes home and starts playing by himself in the street with a paper boat he has made. At six o'clock it starts raining, and he goes inside the house. When Abuelita comes back, he starts talking with her. Abuelita is very happy that Coyote remained close to home playing and did not run away, so that she could find him there. She is also happy that he is such a helpful child, always helpful when she is cooking

> "He can cook mushroom soup, sausages with green chilli, fried chips. Abuelita is proud of him because he plays but he also studies. He is good at maths. He gives a hand to Abuelita, helps her to do the washing up, and does all she asks him to do. Coyote feels very happy with Abuelita. He loves to live with her, he is very fond of Abuelita because when he helps her with the cooking she gives him presents. A toy, or some sweets. . . ."

This idyllic image of an only child reveals Pedro's fantasy of becoming a very special one for Abuelita. In one story the main character talks about what he will do when he is an adult:

> "He is going to buy his own shoes and socks, and even to buy a car. With the car he is going to pick up Abuelita and go for a ride."

This is a very obvious Oedipal phantasy of carrying off his maternal figure in romantic fashion.

Although jealousy is not present in this Oedipal fantasy, there was an important adult in the home, a man called Jorge, who became the object of great jealousy; in Pedro's mind he formed a couple with Bibiana, the house mother.

Very painful feelings of jealousy of the other children are experienced also by Pedro. Abuelita is perceived as having great riches, and Pedro would like to keep everything to himself.

> "It was a Monday morning, it was freezing cold. Taz was eating lots and lots of fruit, which were supposed to be eaten for supper by all the children. He stole them from the fridge. When Abuelita asked for the fruit, Taz told her that they were inside his stomach. Then Abuelita picked some more fruits from one of her fruit trees, and Taz ate even more fruit . . . and Abuelita never gets angry, because when they are short of fruit she can pick more from the fruit tree."

Here we have a real feeling of plenty: Abuelita has so many fruit trees that she can feed the very hungry Taz and there will be enough left for the other children of the children's home. Taz appears here to be again an only child. It is interesting that, in this story, one can see the link between feeling cold, when it rains (when one is sad or cries?), and feeling very hungry. The reference to feeling cold is reminiscent of the story of the "gang hideout" on top of the world, the place where it was very cold. When with Abuelita, he does *not* feel cold. One way that Pedro has to deal with cold in his heart is to eat and eat. Abuelita provides not only warmth but an inexhaustible source of nourishment. The feeling of plenty in the story of the many trees is a good defence against jealousy of the other children. One does not need to be jealous or possessive when there is *so much* to go round. This is, sadly, not the truth of life in a children's home.

At times Pedro is a little more in contact with reality. Jealousy can evoke murderous feelings towards the other children. This is strikingly portrayed symbolically in a story entitled *"El pez Flounder"* [The fish called Flounder]. Before quoting from the story, I would like to note that the containment of Casa Juconi and of "Special Time" enables some of these very traumatized children to move to a symbolic form of expression. This reduces the risk of their being violent with one another.

In the story about Flounder, Pedro tells us about an intriguing fish who apparently gets very tired when they make him go out for walks.

> "Flounder hated walking because he got very tired."

Flounder used to live in a puddle, a rather dirty place, but he liked it. He was then offered a place in a large fish bowl. The problem in this fish bowl was the presence of many other fish.

> "Flounder was frightened . . . when he was frightened, he got into a corner and refused to eat. He tried to dispel his fear by going back to his old home and eating the dirty water of the puddle. Flounder has a dream, that when he will be a big fish he will eat up all the little fish. He will live with Abuelita and help her to do the cooking."

What follows is the dramatic end of the story. There is a jump in time. Flounder has now become a big fish.

> "He gobbles all the little fish and departs with Abuelita. And yes, at the end, no other fish was left. He had exterminated them all."

Here, albeit in fantasy, Pedro has allowed all his most violent feelings and fantasies of exterminating his rivals to come to the fore. No parent is going to interfere with his *omnipotent* destructiveness, and no guilt or regret is experienced.

Pedro's narrative continues through the stories, and gradually we see a change concerning his omnipotence: we had heard in one of the first stories that he could fly up to a planet where he was going to meet his friends from the street.

At that point Pedro was talking about flying and he seemed very sure of his omnipotent capacity. He flew to the planet, to the star he was going to bring to Abuelita, then flew back to the children's home. But in one of the later stories he realizes that he has no wings.

> "What Piolin [the main character] likes about the butterflies is that they fly, and . . . Piolin would like to be like them, he would love to fly, but he cannot because he has no wings."

The lessening of the omnipotence in this story is accompanied by feelings that touch on the anxieties related to damage done and a wish to repair—the anxieties Melanie Klein describes as *depressive* (Klein, 1935). Piolin is annoyed about the impossibility of visiting his natural parents. He is in Abuelita's house, and he smears the walls with toothpaste.

> "Abuelita was cooking and did not realize what was happening. At some point Piolin stopped smearing the walls and immediately started cleaning away the smears all by himself. Abuelita did not reproach him because she never knew what he had done."

The last story in this sequence is a particularly significant one as it conveys the importance of vigilance by a protective parental object. Abuelita must be fully aware that Pedro could be in danger. He might not be strong enough to resist the lure of his old friends, of the dubious company he used to keep in the street. He could ally himself with destructive gang aspects of his internal world. It is not enough for him to say: "I may visit my friends, but I will always come back to Abuelita." He needs to know that he could be rescued, because the gang does not easily let go. This is obviously a reference to the danger that something destructive—much more destructive than smearing toothpaste—may prevail in Pedro over his attraction for the safe, clean fish bowl, the children's home, and the parental figure, Abuelita.

> "One day Piolin was looking for Abuelita. He was in the park and was hiding behind a tree when he encountered a grown-up man he did not know. The man kidnapped Piolin. As he was taking him away, Abuelita saw that he had been kidnapped and rushed to protect him, so they would not take him away. But they also took Abuelita away, to a very large house where lived the 'great one', and left them there. Piolin was very frightened because he did not know what was going to happen. He felt like crying, he didn't feel safe. Then the 'great one' told him that he was going to eat him up.
>
> Piolin said that he would rather be his friend and please not to eat him. But then Abuelita hit the 'great one' with her hand, and Abuelita and Piolin ran away and joined the others at home. When they arrived at the house, they called an extraordinary meeting in order to talk about what had happened and showed everybody that they were safe."

Here the whole story is repeated because Piolin narrates it in some detail to the other children. Having heard the story, the younger ones in the group asked what they should do if something happened to them.

> "Abuelita told them never to go to play in the park and only to play in the garden of the house."

Pedro must have known that this story was an important one, because it is the only one where the narrative is repeated. The grown-up he met behind the tree may well have some links with gang members actually recruiting in the street.

The dynamics I discussed in our meetings are not only related to external aspects of the children's life. The kidnappers may well represent aspects of the child's personality that are drawn to returning to live in the street, to a world of glue sniffing, drug trafficking, and at times prostitution. The Charco—"the puddle"—can be very attractive when the gang, either external or internal, kidnaps and seduces away from good objects a part of the personality. As many psychoanalysts (Joseph, 1982; Meltzer, 1979; Rosenfeld, 1971; Steiner, 1982) have said, it is not easy to escape.

The good object, the parents, Abuelita in the story, may try to retrieve the kidnapped child, but the gang may assert its greater strength, and it may look at times as if the good object may be overcome by it. In Pedro's story Abuelita appears to have succumbed, and Pedro as well is prepared to ally himself with the ring leader, "the great man", the godfather. It is better to be his friend than to be eaten up by him. It is a source of hope that in Pedro's internal world the good objects, the safe home, all that Abuelita stands for, appears to be stronger than the gang. Abuelita just with her hand deals a mighty blow to the head of the godfather.

Pedro knows that the danger is still lurking behind the trees. The frightening story needs to be told and told again. It is as if the fear is still alive in Pedro's mind when he narrates the story, because he ends up by saying that the children should never leave the children's home, just play in the garden.

Discussion

I am always aware when I take work discussion seminars that I am using a large number of psychoanalytic ideas and that I have a psychoanalytic frame of reference. The approach in discussing the material is based on looking at what is observable and formulating some hypotheses on the basis of theories that can be shared without using jargon.

I would like to pinpoint some of the main theories that helped me to understand Pedro's material. I will start with the central theme of his fear of dependence. This is very clear in the first story I mentioned when he tries not to be too soft, not to be a child who likes cuddles. This hardness would be part of what I have referred to as "gang dynamics" (Williams, 1997). The gang might have been in the lives of many of these children an actual experience while they were in the street, but I have also made reference to the presence of an internal gang. This is a concept formulated by Rosenfeld in 1971, but important developments of this concept are to be found in papers by Meltzer (1979), Joseph (1982), and Steiner (1982). The gang is a narcissistic structure that offers protection to a vulnerable part of the self. It is a conglomeration of destructive aspects of the personality that seduce the vulnerable parts into an alliance, promising that there will be no pain and no feeling of need or dependence on parental objects. There will be no feelings of loss because a gang that is internal is, unlike external parents, always present, always available. We see how strong the hold of the gang can be because at the beginning of Pedro's stories, he voluntarily goes to his friends in the place where it is very cold. But after he has made a statement about wanting to stay with

Abuelita, we see that the gang comes back, and there is a real struggle between the menacing and apparently very strong gang structure and Abuelita, representing Pedro's good objects. It looks as if the gang may be stronger. This could be part of what Rosenfeld writes about when he refers to the gang's propaganda, saying "We are the strongest, come with us." It is crucial that in the end Pedro perceives his good object as stronger than the destructive aspects of his personality (the gang). He turns to the vulnerable part of himself by turning to the children in the home and saying, "Look, you are still in danger, look out and keep in a safe place." He is saying this to himself, knowing how strong the temptation is to return to the street, but also to an *internal alliance* with the gang.

This seems to be an impressive development in the limited period of Special Time that this child had, but it is not linear, and there are bound to be fluctuations. We see that he does not want to be dependent, he pushes away the potentially comforting good object (no hugs) but then realizes that without such protection he is going to feel very cold. This theme of "feeling cold" is present in the gang's place on top of the world, and when Pedro is feeling cold, he binges on fruit. His greed is related to the feeling of loneliness. This may be linked to not having as yet firmly established a relationship with a good object and trying to fill the empty space inside with an abundance of food. This topic is explored in some chapters on eating disorders in *The Generosity of Acceptance* (Williams, Williams, Desmarais, Ravenscroft, 2004). There is indeed a great deal of greed in Pedro, not only in terms of food: he would like to have his object all for himself, to be an only child, to be Abuelita's favourite. He tries to protect himself from the fear that his greed might be harmful with the fantasy of the feeling of plenty. The fear of doing harm, which we get only a glimpse of when he smears the wall with toothpaste and then hurries to repair the damage, touches on depressive anxiety as described by Klein when she spoke for the first time of the "depressive position" (Klein, 1935). Other depressive anxieties are present in the story where the children feel sad because the parents do not visit them. When they are in a group, not in a gang, they are able to face feelings of loss. In fact, this is one of the important differences between group dynamics and gang dynamics (Williams, 1997): the gang protects the vulnerable part from being dependent, while the group can think about the absent parents and can thus offer a container. This container does not promise freedom from dependence, as the gang does, but enables psychic pain to be tolerated and strengthens the capacity to withstand addiction to destructiveness. Psychic damage would be present if we saw consistent hardening of the violent aspects of Pedro, as in the story of the fish Flounder, where he devours all the other fish with no feelings of guilt. However, Pedro is not a hardened child and can translate his murderous feelings into a metaphor.

I have described the danger of defences developed by some deprived children in my paper entitled "Doubly Deprived" (Henry, 1974). By "doubly deprived" I meant deprived children who have developed defences and created internal alliances that make it very difficult for them to accept help and make them tie the hands of those trying to help them, thus bringing about a "double deprivation". There are brief moments when Pedro hardens himself using omnipotence as a defence, but the wish to bring a star to Abuelita is far from the state of mind of a hardened child. Pedro seems to find—or perhaps recapture—an experience of a relationship with a precious object worthy of receiving stars as a gift. I find helpful Meltzer's hypothesis (Meltzer, 1988) that every child has the experience of his mother as the most precious creature in the world. We can imagine that such an aesthetic experience might have been present, even if briefly, in Pedro's early days, since a child who responds so well to the offer of help is likely to have had a taste of earlier good experiences. He returned to omnipotent fantasies when he had little containment to rely upon. Indeed, omnipotent fantasies may be a necessary safeguard for children who do not otherwise feel held together by a good object. This predicament has been described very vividly by Joan Symington (1985).

A turning point in the stories is the moment when Pedro realizes that he has no omnipotent powers, that he cannot fly. I remember discussing this lessening of Pedro's omnipotence in the work discussion group in Mexico and linking it with the very significant struggle between the good object and the destructive aspects in the story where both Pedro and Abuelita are kidnapped. The central point of the story is that the vulnerable part does not ally itself with the kidnappers. When he realizes that the good object is stronger, that Abuelita can hit the godfather on the head and can take him away from the gang's hideout, he is certainly relieved, and he engages in trying to save other vulnerable children, and vulnerable parts of himself. It is very important indeed that his story is narrated twice, because Pedro, without having read Rosenfeld, Steiner, Joseph, or Meltzer, knows that the gang does not give up easily!

IV

EPILOGUE

CHAPTER ELEVEN

Work discussion: implications for research and policy

Michael Rustin

The method of work discussion is highly particular—it depends on a single individual practitioner observing himself or herself while actively involved in a work situation and reflecting on the implications of what is being seen and experienced. A work discussion seminar supervises and reflects on each member's observations and reports, and in that way there is a sharing of knowledge and understanding between practitioners whose work situations will usually have something in common. Nevertheless, it is the individual's experience of a situation that is the focus of exploration according to this method.

Work discussion, since its inception, has had two major purposes. The first of these, which it shares with the method of infant observation, is educational and formative. It is intended, like infant observation from whose procedures it derives to a substantial degree, to enhance the psychoanalytic understanding and capacities of those who undertake it, outside or prior to their use by the learner/practitioner in a clinical context. Its usual participants are students engaged in work in educational, health, or care settings who are invited to conduct "participant observations" in their places of work and reflect on them in small seminars originally modelled on those that take place in infant observation programmes. The similarities lie in the method of presentation of detailed observational reports followed by supervisory and peer discussion, in the small scale of the activity (ideally five or so seminar members in a group, permitting two presentations per student in each term), and in its continuity of experience (with participant observations preferably continuing for a year or more). This method has been found to provide an opportunity to observe, reflect on, and learn about the emotional and unconscious aspects of work in these settings, which no other activity comparably provides. This has been a context in which some of the most valuable of contemporary psychoanalytic ideas could be learned in their use, and in their relation to experience, rather than merely "learned about" as abstract concepts. Such complex ideas as those of the relations of containment, the mechanisms of splitting and projective identification, "attacks on linking" (Bion, 1959) and on thought, and the varieties of defences against unconscious anxieties have, through this form of learning, become resources for understanding the dynamics of work-settings where human relationships are central. Just as with infant observation, it is found that a combination of the experience-based learning of work discussion, with some parallel learning of relevant psychoanalytic concepts and theories, enables students to find meaning in emotional and unconscious aspects of their experience and to achieve significant development in their capacity for thoughtful practice. In some educational programmes infant observation, and work discussion, and sometimes young child observation too have been undertaken in parallel, together with a course in psychoanalytic theory. The different balance between reflection and activity called for by these settings is often helpful to the learning process.[1]

For most of its history, the parallel method of infant observation has been conceived as one whose purpose is to develop the observer's capacities for understanding and feeling. While it was recognized early on that the presence of an infant observer was often found to be a good and even helpful experience by the mothers and families being observed, giving help to families was not its purpose. It was families without known problems or risks that were asked to receive an observer—they were requested to help an inexperienced student learn about infancy, not to receive a visitor who was going to advise or teach them. It was quite late in the development of this method that the idea that infant observation might in certain circumstances be given a therapeutic purpose became recognized and its possible use for the support of at-risk families tentatively explored. But it is clearly understood that this more "therapeutic" conception of infant observation is quite distinct from its usual educative purpose and requires both much greater previous experience on the part of observers and a form of supervision whose focus is different from a purely educational one. While attention is given in "normal" infant observation teaching to the emotional experience of the observation by the families—sometimes this reveals that this experience is appreciated by families and is even found helpful by them—it is the student's learning experience that remains the predominant focus in the normal practice of non-interventive infant observation.

But with the method of work discussion, from the start there could never be so clear a distinction between the purpose of learning from the point of view of the student and the practical implications of the learning process for the work-settings that were being observed. The work discussion observers are also participants, often describing and reporting aspects of their own professional practice: in this respect they are unlike the unobtrusive and inactive infant observers who visit a young family. They are invited to choose the situations they wish to discuss in work discussion seminars, and often these are situations selected by participant–observers for the difficulties to which they are felt to give rise, for themselves as well as for others in their workplace. For example, teachers may present reports of their problems in their relationships with troubled children, or of tensions within a staff group; nurses may describe the painfulness of coping with the emotions aroused by distressed patients; care-workers, the anxieties evoked by adolescents for whom they are responsible. Work discussion seminars are often faced with the task not only of understanding what is going on, and the emotions and anxieties that are in play in a situation, but also of actively trying to help a participant–observer to cope better with a situation and, through this, to enable practice to become more thoughtful. There is indeed sometimes an overlap, in the practice of work discussion, between the discussion of observational experience and what is virtually a clinical supervision, since the practical work that is being reported may sometimes have a directly therapeutic aspect, as with art or drama therapists, counsellors, or many other "care practitioners" who work directly with individuals or groups.

The consequence of this "double purpose" of the work discussion method is that it has, from the beginning, been viewed as a way of mapping the emotional and unconscious complexities of work settings and making possible new descriptions of these. This is not merely to facilitate the learning and development of student–observers; it may also have a more external and practical purpose. Participants in work discussion are often already experienced practitioners in their professional field when they enter this learning situation, even if psychoanalytic thinking as such may be new to them. It has therefore been reasonable to hope that a small improvement in the work of a specific work-group, or even a larger institution, might be the outcome even of a single individual's learning experience. As a contribution to professional formation, work discussion has thus come to be seen as a way of improving institutional practices through enhancing the capacities of practitioners and the contributions to understanding that they can make. As a source of descriptions of hitherto neglected dimensions of relational or institutional processes, work discussion has contributed to the understanding of the ways that educational and care systems actually work and has provided new concepts and descriptions for understanding these. The origins of work discussion in work with general practitioners by Michael Balint, referred to earlier in this book, is an early example of the value of a forerunner of this method for understanding a particular field of practice. Work discussion can make a difference through its implications for the work of an individual in an otherwise conventional work setting, but it can also provide the basis for envisaging a new kind of institutional design. In this book, Alison Hall's description of her work as a nurse in a children's ward is an example of the first kind of application, and Simonetta Adamo and her colleagues' chapter on "Parenting a new institution" is an example of the second.

Work discussion is indeed a method whose boundaries are porous and flexible. Those kinds of organizational consultancy that are informed by psychoanalytic thinking have long made use of methods of observation and reflection that are akin to "work discussion". Some of the concepts found most useful in it—for example, the descriptions of institutional defences against anxiety developed in Menzies Lyth's work—had their origin in the practice of organizational consultancy but are learned and reflected on by new generations of practitioner-observers in work discussion settings. The consultation practices reported in *The Unconscious at Work* (Obholzer & Roberts, 1994) and *Working Beneath the Surface* (Huffington & Armstrong, 2004) are often close in their essence to what we describe here. In relation to schooling, Isca Wittenberg's *The Emotional Aspects of Learning and Teaching* (Salzberger-Wittenberg, Williams, & Osborne, 1983) sets out ideas that have become central to the agenda of work discussion for those working in schools and colleges. The approach described in *Organisations Observed* (Hinshelwood & Skogstad, 2000) is also congruent with what we present here. Many professional training and development courses offered at the Tavistock and Portman NHS Foundation Trust, in disciplines that include social work, nursing, organizational consultancy, and educational counselling, have the work discussion method at the core of their curriculum.

Work discussion and research

The question to be explored in this chapter is whether it may be possible to derive implications of a generalizing kind, both for policy and for research, from this method. Might work discussion prove as fertile as infant observation has done, in developing from what has been primarily a method of learning into a source of new understandings of different fields of professional practice? What would it take, in other words, for work discussion to become a method of research?

Researches in different fields are necessarily different and distinct from one another: many errors and confusions arise from presuming or demanding that all research activity should conform to a single template. Researchers differ in what they postulate as their object of study and in the methods of perception and measurement appropriate to them—that is to say, in their implicit ontologies and epistemologies. They differ in the means by which they typically represent or communicate their findings—what Bruno Latour (1987) terms their characteristic "inscription devices". Thus maps are important to geographers, fossil records to palaeontologists, statistical correlations to epidemiologists, social surveys to—some—sociologists, and clinical case studies to psychoanalysts, because of the distinctive attributes of the findings they seek to report and the forms of representation that follow from these attributes. Research fields also have distinctive communities of reception and understanding: their findings are usually addressed primarily to specialists qualified to understand and assess them, and perhaps to practitioners or policy-makers whose work they are intended to inform. The understanding that there is not one science, but many—though with some important shared principles of respect for logic, for impartiality, for evidence, for empirical testability, and for reliability—has been one of the most important insights that have followed from Thomas Kuhn's seminal *The Structure of Scientific Revolutions* (Kuhn, 1962, 2000) and has been adumbrated and extended by a whole generation of subsequent contributors to the sociology of science and technology (Galison & Stump, 1996; Toulmin, 1972).

The field of work discussion, as it is set out in this book, is primarily an application of psychoanalytic ideas and methods to the emotional and unconscious life of individual workers and the organizational settings of work with children and young people. In so far as its orientation is psychoanalytic, its objects of study are unconscious mental and emotional processes. The non-transparency of unconscious processes, to participants but also often in the first instance to observers, gives rise to distinctive observational difficulties. It is, after all, because unconscious mental processes *are* unconscious, and because understanding of them is sometimes resisted by both individuals and institutions, that they are difficult to observe and take account of, yet they may also be potentially powerful and disruptive. It is often *because* of such disruptive and disturbing effects on both individuals and groups that there is sometimes a deep wish to understand them. The need to understand phenomena of this kind provides the essential motivation of the work discussion method as we describe it.[2]

Psychoanalytic methods have evolved over decades as the most powerful means of investigation of this "unconscious" dimension of reality, and the carefully designed and moderated setting of the clinical consulting room has been its primary instrument of observation (Rustin, 2002, 2007). The investigation of the phenomena of the transference, and, more recently, the countertransference, and the discipline of detailed and meticulous descriptive reporting of all that happens in the clinical setting for subsequent reflection and analysis, are its principal investigative resources. Many of the theoretical ideas found most useful in infant observation and work discussion have their origin in discoveries made in the clinical consulting room. The clinical case study has been the primary form of representation, or "inscription device", of this form of investigation. There has been much criticism of the unreliability and "subjectivity" of clinical reports as a source of data (e.g. by Spence, 1983, 1994), though it is now being shown that it is possible to improve on informal clinical methods of analysis of clinical data through more rigorous modes of analysis. It should become possible to achieve higher standards of validity and reliability in developing concepts and theories from such data. But in any case one must keep in mind that the development of the conceptual and theoretical lexicon of psychoanalysis has been a successful one. The power and scope of psychoanalytic explanation has greatly increased during the hundred-year-long history of psychoanalysis, even though to achieve this it has relied for most of its history on the "craft skills" of clinical interpretation of data obtained in the consulting room. These skills have themselves been developed as the field of psychoanalytic study has been extended. (In many if not most fields of knowledge, advances in substantive knowledge have been linked to advances in the techniques by which knowledge is acquired.)

It is to be expected that extensions of psychoanalytic clinical methods, such as those of infant observation, or of work discussion, will share many of the core attributes of this "parent" clinical method. Fundamental to knowledge generation in these organizational and relational settings are the use of detailed descriptive reports, an attitude of respect for particulars, the grounding of theoretical inference in detailed instances, and the testing of interpretative findings through critical reflection by independent participants, which are also central to psychoanalytic clinical methods. And these are indeed the practical disciplines that participants in work discussion (as in infant observation) are expected to learn in the development of their own observational and interpretative capacities.

Where knowledge is primarily advanced through the accumulation of theoretically informed descriptions of situations and through the discovery of "kinds" of phenomena found to share the same characteristics (in psychoanalytic thinking, these may, for example, be pathological states of mind, or psychic defences, or phases of development), systematic comparison between instances is essential. Research based on the case-study method in psychoanalysis has advanced through such a process of comparison between examples, often following the postulation in the psychoanalytic literature of some new or hitherto unrecognized phenomenon, which has then become the focus of further investigation by practitioners. We can trace the development of many of the most significant concepts in psychoanalysis from such a key initial presentation of an original idea, through its exemplification and testing out in many other instances.[3] Sometimes such investigation has taken a relatively organized form, through the practice of clinical workshops that retain a common focus of attention for a lengthy period (M. E. Rustin, 1991). At other times the context of theoretical development has been less visible, either because the work of an individual analyst has been decisive, or because communication between co-workers has been more informal. Generally it has been the case that the procedures of data collection and data analysis that have been followed in the clinical tradition have depended on a high degree of "craft skill" or "practical knowledge" on the part of practitioners rather than on the use of formal protocols, though there are exceptions, and there is now a significant change taking place in the direction of greater formalization of research methods. The development of university doctoral programmes in the psychoanalytic field has been one significant catalyst of this move towards greater methodological accountability.

It has been shown that the method of infant observation, designed originally as an experience of learning, also has potential as a form of psychoanalytic research (Rustin, 2006). The understanding of parent–infant relationships has been enhanced through the findings of infant observers. In particular, the detailed exploration of the idea of "containment" in the mother–baby relationship, and of the probable outcomes of different forms of containment, more and less favourable to development, has become influential in the field of infant mental health and to the psychoanalytic understanding of children and families.

It seems likely that the original development of the container–contained relation drew not only on Bion's seminal inferences from his clinical experience with psychotic patients, but also on the observational and analytic experience of the early pioneers of infant observation, notably Esther Bick. It has been argued that there is scope for a more sustained deployment for purposes of research of the infant observational method, though this would require some change from the conventional "learning" practice of observations mainly of the spectrum of "normally functioning" families undertaken by infant observers with no previous experience of the field.

But the method of work discussion may have an even greater potential than infant observation for use as a method of research. This is because of the significant measure of professional and institutional knowledge that some practitioner–observers bring to this work from the outset—and also because, as practitioners, participants in work discussion are in a situation that enables them to actively explore and test out the hypotheses that they formulate, giving an "action research" dimension to their involvement.[4]

There are examples to be found in this book of new patterns of activity being developed in settings for work with children, whose outcomes are the subject of clear description and even a measure of informal evaluation. Such concepts—such as those of defences against anxiety, organizational splitting mechanisms, containment (or its lack), and benign and malign kinds of group formation (the contrast made by Gianna Williams between gangs and groups, for example)—do valuable explanatory work in descriptions offered here. Concepts like these, and one can add "borderline states of mind" or states of organizational mindlessness, serve as descriptions—even "diagnoses"—that can be seen to be recognizable as what happens when institutions and groups are subject to stress. On the more positive or proactive side is the idea that reflection on emotional experiences can make a difference to the quality of a human service. Indeed, the creation of space for such reflection—whether on a person-to-person (e.g. nurse-to-patient) basis or in a broader institutional setting—is often what these participant–observers try to make possible. Work discussion is the scene of a form of reflection that takes place outside the work context, yet it may also provide a model of reflective interaction that could usefully take place within it. The chapter by Simonetta Adamo and her colleagues describes how "work discussion" has been formative in the design and operation of a new institution, providing a therapeutic form of schooling for adolescents in Naples who were previously wholly absent or excluded from school.

From the point of view of knowledge generation, it is a weakness of the method that the settings whose work is reflected on in work discussion seminars tend to be different from and therefore difficult to directly compare with one another. The contexts observed may depend simply on the accident of where the participants in a work discussion programme are working. There are, however, advantages in seminar participants being able to think together about different settings. They can, for example, learn that key concepts and ways of understanding can have applications well beyond their own personal experience, to situations that might otherwise have seemed to have few similarities. There are certainly some benefits to be gained from work discussion seminars whose members do not come from the same workplace, since this avoids the potential problems of confidentiality and unwanted feedbacks between what takes place in the reflective space of the seminar and what might then have to be dealt with on a daily basis back at work.

But from a research perspective, one can see advantages in varying the common practice of bringing participant observers together from workplaces of different kinds. One can conjecture that more systematic investigation of a particular kind of institutional context—such as hospital wards, classrooms, care homes, social service departments—would proceed more easily if work discussion seminars were made up of members who were all drawn from similar settings, rather than being assembled in a random way. Comparison between observations, and between "experimental initiatives" made within a distinct kind of workplace—such as a school or a prison—could facilitate understanding, just as has the consideration of similar kinds of phenomena done in clinical workshops in child psychotherapy. It would be interesting to compare the outcomes of the work discussion method when it is practised by participants drawn from different institutions with what happens when participants are from the same institutional workplace. The former approach places the main responsibility for learning on the individual participant, the latter requires a group of participants to understand and take responsibility for their interactions not only within the separate space of the work discussion seminar, but also "back home" in their normal workplace. We will only learn more about these different applications of the work discussion method from experience and comparison.

It would assist the generation of knowledge through work discussion if a "lexicon" of the concepts and theories that have been found most productive, and a literature of studies or cases in which such ideas have found applications, were assembled. There is scope, too, for the development of more formalized methods of analysis of the descriptive reports on which work discussion is based. (One option is to make use of the methods of Grounded Theory, appropriately adapted to this task.) In some practitioner-observer settings it might be possible to audio-record and transcribe interactions—such as records of meetings, for example[5]—although often reliance will have to continue to be made on *post-facto* written records. It may certainly be possible to record the proceedings of work discussion seminars themselves, in order better to understand how theoretical inferences are made from observational data. There thus seem to be several ways in which what has hitherto been an informal though meticulous process of data-gathering, transcription, and analysis could become more systematic and accountable.

In order for work discussion to become a recognized and productive location for research, it will need to be developed in this direction. This would be to follow a pattern of development that took place long ago in the clinical practice of psychoanalysis and, more recently, of infant observation. This should make it possible for work discussion to generate sustained and credible descriptions of the interactive processes, conscious and unconscious, that are its primary field of study. There thus seems to be scope for the development of the existing "formative" and "capacity-building" method of work discussion into a method of research the findings of which could demonstrate the explanatory power of a psychoanalytic way of thinking when it is applied "outdoors", in extra-clinical settings.

Such studies, in so far as they remain within the broad parameters of work discussion as it has been described in this book, are likely to be qualitative in their form. There is a different and, of course, important form of research that sets out to test in a statistically robust way the outcomes and effects of different processes. This is the kind of research approach that dominates current discussions about the "evidence base" of professional practice. But before there can be a useful quantitative test of a theoretical formulation, or of a practical intervention, there needs to be a theoretical formulation or design that is interesting enough to be worth the effort and cost of quantitative measurement, on the scale that this usually requires to achieve validity and reliability. But it need not be a problem if, in the early stages of the development of work discussion as a research method, it is seen to belong to the "context of discovery"—a source of generative new ideas—rather than to the "context of validation" of new knowledge—the process of establishing scope, applicability, and, so far as interventions are concerned, cost-effectiveness. The former stage most often precedes the latter in a productive research process.[6]

Work discussion policy, and practice

"Evidence-based policy" and its performance measures

There is a strong emphasis in contemporary government policy-making and implementation on "evidence-based policy". This usually involves establishing measures of current performance of public sector institutions—such as schools, hospitals, university departments—to bring about improvements in performance through clearly specified interventions, whose aims are often formulated as "targets". Alongside this is guidance about practice, such as that provided for clinical services by NICE (the National Institute for Clinical Excellence) about those treatments with the strongest evidence base.

Examples of such performance measures are waiting lists for NHS care, assessed numeracy and literacy scores in primary education, and the time taken to achieve permanent placements for looked-after children. Such measures sometimes come to be regarded as proxies for broader conceptions of service quality. The case that has recently been argued for making cognitive behaviour therapy available as the treatment of choice for adults suffering from depression (Layard, 2005) is based on reported evidence for the remarkable efficacy of this form of therapy—evidence that is, however, disputed, particularly in regard to the more severe and persistent kinds of depressive illness.

There are risks that the adoption of such measures as the criteria by which the performance of institutions will be judged, even when they are inherently reasonable, can have perverse effects, giving undue priority to those dimensions of an institutional task that are amenable to exact measurement, at the expense of other aspects that are more difficult to calibrate but may in reality be more fundamental.[7] "Evidence-based policy" now unfortunately pays little attention to practice-based evidence.

This is even more the case when the aim is not only to set out specific performance criteria to guide managers and practitioners, but also to provide measures for judging the comparative performance of institutions, required to operate in virtual competition with one another, whose outcomes are reported in published league tables.[8] Such competitive outcomes carry with them rewards (such as a lessened liability to inspection, or greater attractiveness to prospective clients or employees) for those deemed more successful, and sanctions (such as intensified regimes of inspection, the removal of managers, or the closure or take-over of whole institutions) for those labelled as less successful. In these cases, selected performance measures come to be perceived as indicators of more general worth or status. While these ratings may represent an incentive for the more successful or advantaged, they may also be demotivating for the less successful and disadvantaged, increasing rather than decreasing disparities of performance between institutions and their client populations. Preoccupation with the outcomes of such competitive judgement may certainly divert practitioners, and perhaps their clients too, from the primary goals of the services in question, substituting extraneous for intrinsic measures of quality. Sometimes, in fact, the organizational climate that emerges in response to anxieties about meeting prescribed targets worsens the quality of what is provided.

In seeking methods of defining performance in terms that lend themselves to measurement, the application of rewards and sanctions, and the creation of regimes of competition, "the new public management" (Clarke, Gewirtz, & McLaughlin, 2000) has been seeking to find proxies for the largely standardized and replicable measures of turnover and profit that are regulative in market competition. The aim is to find a way of translating qualities into quantities, so to speak, just as financial accounting translates the qualities of supermarkets, theatre performances, or novels, into sales figures and, ultimately, into profit measures. The purpose of such performance criteria may be to find the nearest feasible equivalent to an accountable bottom line that is represented by the balance sheet of a firm in the market. Of course, in addition to these measures of service quality or user satisfaction, financial balance sheets have become critical measures of performance in public sector institutions. Since these institutions are often now located in various kinds of quasi-markets (for patients, students, placements, etc.) and incomes often follow "customer choice" between service providers, equivalents to market regimes within the public sector have widely been created. Since it is desirable that public services *should* improve and that managers and users should to be able to compare the performance of different providers, such forms of measurement seem to be necessary. Without common measures, it is difficult to make meaningful comparisons.

Something, however, that preoccupies many workers in public services, especially those in which human relationships make an important contribution to the quality of a service, is whether performance indicators of this kind adequately measure the quality of a service. They are often believed to leave out of account some of the most important dimensions of the experience of the clients of services, and of those who deliver them. It is to these "missing areas" that the methods of work discussion usually address themselves.

Relationships in work settings

Reflective work discussion, and the kinds of work practices and sensitivities it seeks to enhance, has a conception of interpersonal work, especially in the caring and educational services to which it is most often applied, which contrasts with a dominant managerial focus on measurable targets and outcomes, while not necessarily disputing the usefulness of these. Its emphasis is on the human relationships within which these kinds of work take place, and on the quality of interactions and communication that take place in work-settings. Its particular interest is in the unconscious emotional dynamics that are inseparable from many work situations, especially in the domains of education, health, and welfare.

The guiding assumption of this method of learning is that the provision[9] of human services nearly always takes place in the context of a significant relationship between provider and client. The relationships between teachers and pupils, doctors and nurses and patients, social workers and clients, policemen and citizens whose behaviour they are seeking to keep within acceptable bounds, are examples of such kinds of relationships. There can be no good delivery of human services without a relationship capable of holding and giving appropriate meaning to what is being provided.

As we have suggested earlier, work discussion has been conceived since its inception as an intervention intended to improve professional work. This purpose arises from its fundamental conceptions. These include the idea that high-quality work in the educational, health, and caring fields has a crucial "relational" dimension, and that the "holding in mind" of intense states of feeling is a precondition of good institutional practice. To achieve this, the capacity to relate in understanding and sensitive ways to patients, pupils, clients, and colleagues and to be able to bear the stresses of occupational anxiety need to be developed by individuals, as well as nurtured by the right kinds of supervision and management. Work discussion aims to develop these human capacities, and its advocates believe that such development can lead to broader changes in occupational practice, often in a local way, but sometimes more broadly if there is receptiveness to these approaches within a larger institutional setting or occupational tradition.

Holding in mind

The work discussion method, as noted earlier, has been strongly influenced by the psychoanalytic conception of containment developed by Wilfred Bion and others. The development of the personality in infancy depends, according to this account, on relationships in which the intense feelings and anxieties that are an inescapable part of human growth can be adequately recognized, borne, and understood. Bion's account and Winnicott's parallel one holds that such feelings are, when all goes well, "processed for" the growing infant by its mother or carer, enabling the infant not to be overwhelmed by them. Where an adequate quality of containment is not available, or where care takes actively invasive or harmful forms, anxieties rise to an abnormally high level, and defences may be created to deal with these which are ultimately damaging to emotional development and the capacity to sustain relationships in which love and trust predominate.

The theoretical perspective that underlies the method of work discussion has extended the conception of containment explored systematically in infant observation in the relationships of early infancy to broader contexts of relationship outside the family. Intense emotions and anxieties, explicit or latent, conscious or unconscious, pervade the relationships that individuals form with the institutions on which they depend in significant areas of their lives. Wherever individuals find themselves reliant on the attention and care of others for their well-being, the potential for intense emotion and anxiety will be evoked and may become a dynamic if often unrecognized aspect of a work situation. Some of the practice observations in this book describe relationships between "service providers" and "users" in which a considerable intensity of feeling, need, or desire has been invested. This is different from work situations in which more short-term or casual exchanges between relative strangers are the norm, as in many kinds of commerce or official setting, though we know that these can also evoke strong and anxious feelings when they take an unexpected turn.

Relationships between colleagues at work can also have this dimension. The workplace is a major source of many individuals' identity and sense of worth, and of their ongoing human connectedness.[10] This is the case whether or not the primary task of an organization in which individuals work is concerned with relationships of care. Some of the insights to be derived from the work discussion method are therefore likely to be applicable to work situations of all kinds.

One of the beneficial outcomes of work discussion as a method of learning is to enhance practitioners' capacities to observe and respond in sensitive ways to emotionally charged and complex situations. Practitioner–observers with this experience learn to notice and take in what would formerly have passed them by. They learn more tolerance of unavoidably painful situations and become better able to understand the pain and anger of those they are working with. They become more likely to see constructive and creative solutions to apparent *impasses* in work with clients or colleagues and less likely to respond by flight or by countering aggression with aggression. The case studies in this volume show many examples of such thoughtful and creative responses to work situations full of difficulty.

What can be learned from work discussion?

How, then, might work discussion become a means of improving professional practice and policy-making, aside from its desirable use as part of "continuing professional development" or CPD programmes?

How can this method of "learning from particulars" come to have a broader influence?

It is clear that making available fuller and better documented descriptions of institutional contexts and practices from reports based on the work discussion method can enhance understanding. Such accounts, as seen in this book, can provide compelling evidence, especially when they give meaning and shape to the experience of the providers or users of the services they describe. One should recall that different forms of knowledge usually have not only their distinctive objects and methods, but also their distinctive communities of reception. The communities of reception in the case of work discussion include practitioner communities as well as the larger public, as much as specialists in the social and psychological sciences.

It is important to note that the kinds of research that have a lasting influence are not always those that depend on the quantitative scale of a demonstration. As Rom Harré (1993) has pointed out in his defence of "intensive" in contrast to "extensive" methods in the human sciences, even in the natural sciences much investigation has proceeded from the study of particular instances, by which, as in a crucial experiment, a broader theoretical conception is put to the test. Darwin's discovery, high up on mountain-sides, of the fossilized remains of creatures that must once have lived in the sea was compelling evidence of a process of evolution over time, even when only a few such fossils had been discovered. It only needs the demonstration that *one* species can live and reproduce miles beneath the sea, in the absence of any light from the sun but taking its necessary energy from deep-sea volcanic action, to refute the idea that *all* living creatures depend on solar energy. The distresses and disturbances of quite small numbers of young children, deprived of the proximity of their parents or other familiar carers in hospitals or removed from any attentive care in orphanages, once gave ample evidence of what young children need to thrive. In the latter case, the "inscription device" of documentary films (those of James and Joyce Robertson) were powerful additions to the observed and written-up study of what had happened to the children. And it appears that the observation of the autistic behaviour of children abandoned in neglectful nurseries in Romania has been taken as decisive evidence against an exclusively genetic explanation of autism.

But while numbers are not always decisive—in the first instance, at least—the accuracy and perceptiveness of a description, and its being framed in concepts that name what is essential, is. We might hope that quite small-scale studies based on practitioner–observer experience could change our understanding of work situations and their needs, if they were well-enough focused and described.

There is scope for the work discussion method to have some influence on institutional design too, but in this respect we are at a fairly early stage of development. For this, the conditions for a more systematic approach to institutional research need to be met, including the engagement of more experienced researcher–practitioners, a focus on selected contexts of work—such as day nurseries, infant schools, children's wards, university classes, remand centres—and more accountable methods of data collection and analysis.[11] Demonstrating the value of a psychoanalytically informed approach to institutional practices—the underlying commitment of work discussion—depends on the generation of compelling descriptions of the differences between institutions and practices that *are* able to reflect with understanding on the functions of emotions, relationships, and anxieties and those that are not. Several descriptions of this kind are offered in this book, and we hope that many more will follow.

Notes

1. A broader discussion of the various linked components of the "Tavistock method" of learning from experience can be found in Rustin, 2003.

2. "Work discussion" as described here has a predominantly psychoanalytic focus of interest. It does seem likely, however, that the method of close participative observation of work settings, with regular supervised peer discussion of reported observations, could be undertaken from other disciplinary perspectives—for example, those informed by sociological or anthropological conceptions. Observational methods with a more pedagogic focus have long had an important role in teacher education and professional development, where they have also been assigned a research purpose (a summary with a useful bibliography can be found in Blythman & Macleod, 1989; Hammersley, 1993, explores research issues). What the observation method, and especially work discussion, usually encourages is a process of learning inductively from particular situations, drawing on definite conceptual and theoretical resources as sources of meaning and connection, while still allowing individual experience its own interpretative freedom. There are ways of understanding psychosocial and institutional interactions other than those captured by psychoanalysis that could be developed by this participant observational technique.

3. On the development of psychoanalytic knowledge—mainly in the United Kingdom—from this perspective see Rustin, 2007, 2008, and Judith M. Hughes, 2004.

4. A significant difference between clinical practice and infant observation

from the point of view of research is the opportunity that clinical practice affords for analysts to be active in exploring conjectures and hypotheses, through interpretations and the understanding of what comes of them in a session. By contrast, the largely passive role prescribed for infant observers precludes them from such active exploration in their observation setting (Rustin, 2006). Work discussion lies somewhere between these two methods in this respect.

5. Two doctoral researchers in social work at the Tavistock Clinic, Philippe Mandin and Vimala Uttarkar, are making use of such recordings in their work.

6. On contexts of discovery and validation, see Rudner, 1966.

7. Such diversionary or perverse effects have been pointed out in critiques of contemporary audit systems, for example in Power, 1994; Rustin, 2004; Strathern, 2000; Travers, 2007.

8. Sometimes, in an act of official hypocrisy, the "league tables" are held to be the responsibility of press reporting rather than the audit process itself, even though everyone knows that it is these tables that have the most significant consequences for institutions.

9. More widely used these days is the concept of "service delivery", whose function is to impose a mode of thinking appropriate to commodity distribution onto transactions in which relationships are usually a primary consideration, rather than a secondary one, as they are in transactions in a supermarket.

10. On the changing relationships of work, see Richard Sennett, 2000, 2006.

11. Ongoing work for professional doctorates being undertaken at the Tavistock and Portman NHS Trust in Social Work, Child Psychotherapy, Systemic Therapy, and Organisational Consultancy currently involves studies in several of these settings.

REFERENCES AND BIBLIOGRAPHY

Abrahamsen, G. (1993). The necessary interaction. In: L. Gomnaes & E. Osborne (Eds.), *Making Links: How Children Learn*. Oslo, Norway: Yrkeslitteratur.

Adamo, A., & Rustin, M. (Eds.). (2001). Young child observation. *International Journal of Infant Observation, 4* (2, Special Issue).

Adamo, S. M. G., Adamo Serpieri, S., Giusti, P., Tamajo Contarini, R., & Valerio, P. (2005). The Chance Project: Complex intervention with adolescent school drop-outs in Naples. *Psychodynamic Practice, 11*(3): 239–254.

Adamo, S. M. G., & Aiello, A. (2006). Desperately trying to get through: Establishing contact in work with adolescent drop-outs. *International Journal on School Disaffection, 4* (1): 27–38.

Adamo, S. M. G., Iannazzone, R., Melazzini, C., & Peyron, C. (2005). On not being able to learn: An experimental project for adolescent drop-outs. *Ricerche di Psicologia, 28* (1): 85–110.

Adamo Serpieri, S., & Giusti, P. (2007). Education on the road: Working with adolescent drop-outs in an experimental project. *International Journal on School Disaffection, 5* (1): 11–15.

Adamo Serpieri, S., Giusti, P., Portanova, F., & Tamajo, R. (2003). La bottega del mercoledì. Il lavoro psicologico in moduli territoriali. In: S. M. G. Adamo & P. Valerio (Eds.), *Il contributo psicoanalitico ad una scuola per adolescenti drop-out*. Rome: Grafica Editore Romana.

Ali, E., & Jones, C. (2000). *Report for Camden LEA on the underachievement of Somali pupils*. London: Institute of Education, London University.

Alvarez, A. (1992). *Live Company: Psychoanalytic Psychotherapy with Autistic, Borderline, Deprived and Abused Children*. London: Routledge.

Balint, M. (1957). *The Doctor, His Patient and the Illness*. London: Pitman Medical.

Bennathan, M., & Boxall, M. (1996). *Effective Intervention in Primary Schools: Nurture Groups*. London: David Fulton.

Bernstein, B. (1975). *Class, Codes and Control, Vol. 3: Towards a Theory of Educational Transmissions*. London: Routledge & Kegan Paul.

Bhui, K., Mohamud, S., Warta, N., Stansfeld, S. A., Thornicroft, G., Curtis, S., & McCrone, P. (2006). Mental disorders among Somali refugees: Developing culturally appropriate measures and assessing sociocultural risk factors. *Social Psychiatry and Psychiatric Epidemiology, 41*: 5.

Bick, E. (1968). The experience of skin in early object relations. *British Journal of Psycho-Analysis, 49*, 484–486. Reprinted in: M. Harris Williams (Ed.), *Collected Papers of Martha Harris and Esther Bick*. Strath Tay: Clunie Press, 1989. Also reprinted in: A. Briggs (Ed.), *Surviving Space: Papers on Infant Observation* (pp. 55–59). Tavistock Clinic Series. London: Karnac, 2002.

Bion, W. R. (1959). Attacks on linking. *International Journal of Psycho-Analysis, 40*: 308–15. Reprinted in: W. R. Bion, *Second Thoughts*. London: Heinemann, 1967; reprinted London: Karnac, 1993.

Bion, W. R. (1961). *Experiences in Groups and Other Papers*. London: Routledge.

Bion, W. R. (1962a). *Learning from Experience*. London: Heinemann; reprinted London: Karnac, 1984.

Bion, W. R. (1962b). A theory of thinking. *International Journal of Psycho-Analysis, 43*: 306–310.

Bion, W. R. (1963). *Elements of Psychoanalysis*. London: Heinemann.

Bion, W. R. (1965). *Transformations*. London: Karnac, 1984.

Bion, W. R. (1967a). Attacks on linking. In: *Second Thoughts*. London: Heinemann; reprinted London: Karnac.

Bion, W. R. (1967b). *Second Thoughts*. London: Heinemann; reprinted London: Karnac.

Bion, W. R. (1970). *Attention and Interpretation*. London: Tavistock.

Bion, W. R. (1997). *Taming Wild Thoughts*. London: Karnac.

Blythman, M., & MacLeod, D. (1989). *Classroom Observation from Inside. Spotlights, 16*. Scottish Council for Research in Education. Available at scre.ac.uk/pdf/spotlight/spotlight16.pdf

Boston, M. (1983). Technical problems in therapy. In: M. Boston & R. Szur (Eds.), *Psychotherapy with Severely Deprived Children*. London: Routledge.

Boston, M., & Szur, R. (1969). *Psychotherapy with Severely Deprived Children*. London: Routledge & Kegan Paul.

Bourne, S. (1981). *Under the Doctor: Studies in the Psychological Problems of Physiotherapists, Patients and Doctors*. Amersham: Avebury.

Bowlby, J. (1969). *Attachment and Loss, Vol. I*. London: Hogarth Press.

Bowlby, J. (1973). *Attachment and Loss, Vol. II*. London: Hogarth Press.

Bowlby, J. (1979). On knowing what you are not supposed to know and feeling what you are not supposed to feel. In: *A Secure Base: Clinical Applications of Attachment Theory*. London: Routledge, 1997.

Bowlby, J. (1980). *Attachment and Loss, Vol. III*. London: Hogarth Press.

Bradley, J. (1991). Finding room for thought: A struggle against mindless conflict. In: S. M. G. Adamo & G. Polacco Williams (Eds.), *Working with Disruptive Adolescents*. Naples: Monografie dell'Istituto Italiano degli Studi Filosofici, 11.

Bradley, J. (1997). *How the Patient Informs the Process of Supervision: The Patient as Catalyst*. In: G. Shipton (Ed.), *Supervision of Psychotherapy and Counselling*. Milton Keynes: Open University Press.

Briggs, A. (Ed.) (2002). *Surviving Space*. Tavistock Clinic Series. London: Karnac.

Briggs, S., & Canham, H. (1999). Editorial. *International Journal of Infant Observation, 2* (2). [Special Edition on Observation and Social Work.]

Brook, P. (1998). *Threads of time: A Memoir*. London: Methuen Drama.

Bruner, J. S., Jolly, A., & Sylva, K. (Eds.) (1976). *Play: Its Role in Development and Evolution*. Harmondsworth: Penguin.

Canham, H. (1999). The development of time and space in fostered and adopted children. *Psychoanalytic Inquiry, 19* (2): 160–171.

Canham, H. (2002). Group and gang states of mind. *Journal of Child Psychotherapy, 28* (2): 113–127.

Cifali, M. (1994). *Le lien éducatif. Contre-jour psychanalytique*. Paris: Presses Universitaires de France.

Clarke, J., Gewirtz, S., & McLaughlin, E. (Eds.) (2000). *New Managerialism, New Welfare?* London: Sage.

Claxton, G. (2003). *Creativity: A Guide for the Advanced Learner (and Teacher)*. Bristol: University of Bristol, Graduate School of Education.

Coleridge, S. T. (1817). *Biographia Literaria*. Available at www.gutenberg.org/etext/6081.

Copley, B. (1993). *The World of Adolescence: Literature, Society and Psychoanalytic Psychotherapy*. London: Free Association Books.

Copley, B., & Forryan, B. (1997). *Therapeutic Work with Children and Young People.* London: Cassell; London: Redwood Books.

Davenhill, R., Balfour, A., & Rustin, M. (2007). Psychoanalytic observation and old age. In: R. Davenhill (Ed.), *Looking into Later Life.* Tavistock Clinic Series. London: Karnac.

DfES/DoH (November 2006). *Report on the Implementation of Standard 9 of the National Service Framework for Children, Young People and Maternity Services. Annex: Models of Good Practice.* London: Department for Education and Skills/Department of Health.

Dollery, J. (2002). *Secondary Skin and Culture: Reflections on Some Aspects of Teaching Traveller Children.* In: A. Briggs (Ed.), *Surviving Space.* Tavistock Clinic Series. London: Karnac.

Douglas, M. (1970) *Natural Symbols: Explorations in Cosmology.* London: Cresset Press.

Egeland, B., & Susman-Stillman, A. (1996). Dissociation as a mediator of child abuse across generations. *Child Abuse and Neglect, 20*: 1123–1132.

Fox, M. (1995). Working to support refugees in schools. In: J. Trowell & M. Bower (Eds.), *The Emotional Needs of Young Children and Their Families.* London: Routledge.

Freud, S. (1895d). *Studies on Hysteria.* In: *Standard Edition, 2.*

Freud, S. (1915a). Observations on transference love. In: *Standard Edition, 12.* London: Hogarth Press.

Freud, S. (1917e [1915]). Mourning and melancholia. In: *Standard Edition, 14.* London: Hogarth Press.

Friedman, L. (1982). "The Interplay of Evocation." Paper presented at the Postgraduate Centre for Mental Health, New York.

Furman, E. (1984). Helping children cope with dying. *Journal of Psychotherapy, 10.*

Galison, P., & Stump, D. J. (Eds.) (1996). *The Disunity of Science.* Stanford, CA: Stanford University Press.

Glaser, B. G. (1992). *Basics of Grounded Theory Analysis: Emergence vs Forcing.* Mill Valley, CA: Sociology Press.

Glaser, B. G., & Strauss, A. L. (1967). *The Discovery of Grounded Theory: Strategies for Qualitative Research.* Chicago: Aldine.

Guerin, B., Guerin, P. B., Diiriye, R. O., & Yates, S. (2004). Somali conceptions and expectations concerning mental health: Some guidelines for mental health professionals. *New Zealand Journal of Psychology, 33* (2, July).

Hammersley, M. (Ed.) (1993). *Controversies in Classroom Research.* Milton Keynes: Open University Press.

Hardiman, P. S., & Lapeyre, F. (2004). *Youth and Exclusion in Disadvantaged Urban Areas: Policy Approaches in Six European Cities. Trends in Social Cohesion 9*. Strasbourg: Council of Europe Publishing.

Harré, R. (1993). *Social Being* (2nd edition). London: Blackwell.

Harris, M. (1987). Bion's conception of a psycho-analytical attitude. In: M. Harris Williams (Ed.), *Collected Papers of Martha Harris and Esther Bick*. London: Karnac.

Hartland-Rowe, L. (2005). Teaching and observing in work discussion. In: *International Journal of Infant Observation, 8* (1).

Henry, G. (1974). Doubly deprived. *Journal of Child Psychotherapy, 3* (4): 29–43. Reprinted in: G. Williams, *Internal Landscapes and Foreign Bodies*. London: Duckworth, 1997.

Hinshelwood, R. D. (1998). *A Dictionary of Kleinian Thought*. London: Free Association Books.

Hinshelwood, R. D. (2002). Applying the observational method: Observing organisations. In: A. Briggs (Ed.), *Surviving Space: Papers on Infant Observation* (pp. 157–171). Tavistock Clinic Series. London: Karnac.

Hinshelwood, R. D., & Skogstad, W. (Eds.) (2000). *Observing Organisations: Anxiety, Defence and Culture in Health Care*. London: Routledge.

Hinshelwood, R. D., & Skogstad, W. (2002). Irradiated by distress: Observing psychic pain in health-care organisations. *Psychoanalytic Psychotherapy, 16* (2): 110–124.

Hopkins, J. (1986). Solving the mystery of monsters: Steps towards the recovery from trauma. *Journal of Child Psychotherapy, 12* (1): 61–72.

Hopkins, J. (1990). The observed infant of attachment theory. In: *British Journal of Psychotherapy, 6*: 460–471.

Hoxter, S. (1981). La vecchia donna che viveva in una scarpa [The old woman who lived in a shoe]. In: S. M. G. Adamo (Ed.), *Il Progetto Chance. Seminari psicologici*. Rome: Grafica Editrice Romana.

Huffington, C., & Armstrong, D. (Eds.) (2004). *Working Beneath the Surface: The Emotional Life of Contemporary Organisations*. London: Karnac.

Hughes, J. M. (2004). *From Obstacle to Ally: The Making of Psychoanalytic Practice*. Hove: Brunner-Routledge.

Irvine, E. (1959). The use of small group discussions in the teaching of human relations and mental health. *British Journal of Psychiatric Social Work, 5*.

Jackson, E. (2002). Mental health in schools: What about the staff? *Journal of Child Psychotherapy, 28* (2): 129–146.

Jackson, E. (2005). Developing observation skills in school settings: The importance and impact of "work discussion groups" for staff. *International Journal of Infant Observation, 8* (1): 5–17.

Jackson, E. (2008). The development of work discussion groups in educational settings. *Journal of Child Psychotherapy, 34* (1): 62–82.

Johnston, D. (1992). *Children of Offenders*. Pasadena, CA: Pacific Oaks Centre for Children of Incarcerated Parents.

Joseph, B. (1982). Addiction to near death. *International Journal of Psycho-Analysis, 63*: 449–456.

Judd, D. (1995). *Give Sorrow Words: Working with a Dying Child*. London: Whurr.

Kahin, M. H. (1998) Somali children: The need to work in partnership with parents and community. *Multicultural Teaching, 17*.

Klein, M. (1923). The role of school in the libidinal development of the child. In: *Love, Guilt and Reparation and Other Works 1921–1945* (pp. 59–76). London: Hogarth Press, 1975; London: Vintage, 1998.

Klein, M. (1927). Criminal tendencies in normal children. In: *Love, Guilt and Reparation and Other Works 1921–1945* (pp. 170–185). London: Hogarth Press, 1975; London: Vintage, 1998.

Klein, M. (1928). Early stages of the Oedipus Conflict. In: *Love, Guilt and Reparation and Other Works 1921–1945* (pp. 186–198). London: Hogarth Press, 1975; London: Vintage, 1998.

Klein, M. (1930). The importance of symbol formation in the development of the ego. In: *Love, Guilt and Reparation and Other Works 1921–1945* (pp. 219–232). London: Hogarth Press, 1975; London: Vintage, 1998.

Klein, M. (1931). A contribution of the theory of intellectual development. In: *Love, Guilt and Reparation and Other Works 1921–1945* (pp. 236–248). London: Hogarth Press, 1975; London: Vintage, 1998.

Klein, M. (1935). A contribution to the psychogenesis of manic-depressive states. In: *Love, Guilt and Reparation and Other Works 1921–1945* (pp. 262–289). London: Hogarth Press, 1975; London: Vintage, 1998.

Klein, M. (1937). Love, guilt and reparation. In: *Love, Guilt and Reparation and Other Works 1921–1945* (pp. 306–343). London: Hogarth Press, 1975; London: Vintage, 1998.

Klein, M. (1940). Mourning and its relation to manic-depressive states. In: *Love, Guilt and Reparation and Other Works 1921–1945* (pp. 344–369). London: Hogarth Press 1975; London: Vintage, 1998.

Klein, M. (1946). Notes on some schizoid mechanisms. In: *Envy and Gratitude and Other Works 1946–1963* (pp. 1–24). London: Hogarth Press 1975; London: Vintage, 1997.

Klein, M. (1959). Our adult world and its roots in infancy. In: *Envy and Gratitude and Other Works 1946–1963* (pp. 247–263). London: Hogarth Press, 1975; London: Vintage, 1997.

Klein, M. (1961). *Narrative of a Child Analysis*. London: Vintage, 1998.

Klein, M. (1975). *Envy and Gratitude and Other Works 1946–1963.* London: Hogarth Press.

Kuhn, T. S. (1962). *The Structure of Scientific Revolutions.* Chicago: Chicago University Press.

Kuhn, T. S. (2000). *The Road Since Structure: Philosophical Essays 1970–1990, with an Autobiographical Interview*, ed. J. Conant & J. Haugeland. Chicago: Chicago University Press.

Landy, R. (1993). *Person and Performance.* London: Jessica Kingsley.

Lanyado, M. (1985). Surviving trauma: Dilemmas in the psychotherapy of traumatised children. *British Journal of Psychotherapy, 2* (1): 50–62.

Lanyado, M. (2001). Daring to try again: The hope and pain of forming new attachments. *Therapeutic Communities, 22* (1): 5–18.

Lapeyre, F. (2004). Case study of the *Quartieri Spagnoli* (Spanish quarter) of Naples, Italy: Analyses and recommendations based on the experience of the Chance Project. In: P. S. Hardiman & F. Lapeyre, *Youth and Exclusion in Disadvantaged Urban Areas: Policy Approaches in Six European Cities. Trends in Social Cohesion.* Strasbourg: Council of Europe Publishing.

Latour, B. (1987). *Science in Action: How to Follow Scientists and Engineers through Society.* Milton Keynes: Open University Press.

Layard, R. (2005). *Happiness: Lessons from a New Science.* London: Allen Lane/Penguin.

Lopez-Corvo, R. E. (2003). *The Dictionary of the Work of W. R. Bion.* London: Karnac.

Lyons-Ruth, K., & Block, D. (1996). The disturbed caregiving system: Relations among childhood trauma, maternal caregiving, and infant affect and attachment. *Infant Mental Health Journal, 17*: 257–275.

Magliulo, M. F. (2003). *Vermi solitari, pulci, vulcani e "pietre pomici". Una lezione di scienze a chance* [Solitary worms, fleas, volcanoes, and "pumice stones". A science lesson at chance]. In: S. M. G. Adamo & P. Valerio (Eds.), *Il contributo psicoanalitico ad una scuola per adolescenti drop-out.* Rome: Grafica Editrice Romana.

Main, M., & Goldwyn, R. (1984). Predicting rejection of her infant from mother's representation of her own experience: Implications for the abused–abusing generational cycle. *Child Abuse and Neglect, 8*: 203–217.

Meltzer, D. (1979). *Sexual States of Mind.* Strath Tay: Clunie Press.

Meltzer, D. (1988). *The Apprehension of Beauty.* Strath Tay: Clunie Press.

Meltzer, D., & Harris, M. (1986). Family patterns and cultural educability. In: D. Meltzer (Ed), *Studies in Extended Metapsychology.* Strath Tay: Clunie Press.

Menzies, I. (1959). The functioning of social systems as a defence against anxiety. In: I. Menzies Lyth, *Containing Anxiety in Institutions, Selected Papers, Vol. 1*. London: Free Associations Books, 1988.

Menzies Lyth, I. (1985). The development of the self in children in institutions. In: J. Trowell & M. Bower (Eds.), *The Emotional Needs of Young Children and Their Families: Using Psychoanalytic Ideas in the Community*. London: Routledge.

Menzies Lyth, I. (1988). *Containing Anxiety in Institutions: Selected Essays, Vols. 1 & 2*. London: Free Association Books.

Menzies Lyth, I. (1997). *Containing Anxiety in Institutions: Selected Essays: Vol. 1*. London: Free Associations Books.

Miller, E., & Rice, A. K. (1967). *Systems of Organisation: The Control of Task and Sentient Boundaries*. London: Tavistock Publications.

Miller, L., Rustin, M., Rustin, M., & Shuttleworth, J. (Eds.) (1989). *Closely Observed Infants*. London: Duckworth.

Money-Kyrle, R. (1956). Normal counter-transference and some of its deviations. In: D. Meltzer (Ed.), *The Collected Papers of Roger Money-Kyrle*. Strath Tay: Clunie Press, 1978.

Money-Kyrle, R. (1977). Success and failure in mental maturations. D. Meltzer (Ed.), *The Collected Papers of Roger Money-Kyrle* (pp. 397–432). Strath Tay: Clunie Press, 1978.

Negri, R. (1994). *The Newborn in the Intensive Care Unit*. London: Karnac.

Obholzer, A., & Roberts, V. Z. (Eds.) (1994). *The Unconscious at Work*. London: Routledge.

Oliva, S. (1987). Note sull'osservazione psicoanalitica secondo W. Bion. In: C. Neri, A. Correale, & P. Fadda (Eds.), *Letture bioniane*. Rome: Borla.

O'Shaughnessy, E. (1964). The absent object. *Journal of Child Psychotherapy, 1* (2): 34–43.

Power, M. (1994). *The Audit Explosion*. London: Demos.

Reid, S. (Ed.). (1997). *Developments in Infant Observation*. London: Routledge.

Rice, A. K. (1963). *The Enterprise and Its Environment*. London: Tavistock.

Robertson, J. (1958). *Young Children in Hospital*. London: Tavistock.

Rosenfeld, H. (1971). A clinical approach to the psychoanalytical theory of the life and death instincts: An investigation into the aggressive aspects of narcissism. *International Journal of Psychoanalysis, 52*: 169–178.

Rudner, R. (1966). *Philosophy of Social Science*. Englewood Cliffs, NJ: Prentice-Hall.

Rustin, M. E. (1989). Foreword. In: L. Miller, M. E. Rustin, M. J. Rustin, & J. Shuttleworth, *Closely Observed Infants*. London: Duckworth.

Rustin, M. E. (1991). The strengths of a practitioner's workshop as a new model in clinical research, In: S. Miller & R. Szur (Eds.), *Extending Horizons*. London: Karnac.

Rustin, M. J. (2002). Give me a consulting room: The generation of psychoanalytical knowledge. In: *Reason and Unreason*. London: Continuum.

Rustin, M. J. (2003). Learning about emotions: The Tavistock approach. *European Journal of Psychotherapy, Counselling and Health, 6* (3), 187–208.

Rustin, M. J. (2004). Rethinking audit and inspection. *Soundings, 26* (Spring): 86–107.

Rustin, M. J. (2006). Infant observation research: What have we learned so far? *Infant Observation, 9* (1): 35–52.

Rustin, M. J. (2007). How do psychoanalysts know what they know? In: L. Braddock & M. Lacewing (Eds.), *The Academic Face of Psychoanalysis*. London: Routledge.

Rustin, M. J. (2008). What do child psychotherapists know? In: N. Midgley, J. Anderson, T. Nesic-Vuckovic, & C. Urwin (Eds.), *Child Psychotherapy and Research: New Approaches, Emerging Findings*. London: Routledge.

Salavou, V., Jackson, E., & Oddy, P. (2002). *Brent Secondary Schools Needs Assessment Project*. London: Brent Centre for Young People.

Salmon, G. (1993). The link between the end and the beginning in education therapy. In: L. Gomnaes & E. Osborne (Eds.), *Making Links: How Children Learn*. Oslo: Yrkeslitteratur.

Salzberger-Wittenberg, I., Henry, G., & Osborne, E. (1983). *The Emotional Experience of Learning and Teaching*. London: Routledge & Kegan Paul.

Salzberger-Wittenberg, I., Williams G., & Osborne, E. (1983). *The Emotional Aspects of Learning and Teaching*. London: Routledge; reprinted London: Karnac, 1999.

Segal, H. (1964). *Introduction to the Work of Melanie Klein*. New York: Basic Books.

Sennett, R. (2000). *The Corrosion of Character: The Personal Consequences of Work in the New Capitalism*. New York: W. W. Norton.

Sennett, R. (2006). *The Culture of the New Capitalism*. New Haven, CT: Yale University Press.

Shweder, R. A., & Bourne, E. J. (1984). Does the concept of the person vary cross-culturally? In: R. A. Shweder & R. A. Levine (Eds.), *Culture Theory: Essay on Mind, Self and Emotion*. Cambridge: Cambridge University Press.

Sinason, V. (1992). *Mental Handicap and the Human Condition: New Approaches from the Tavistock*. London: Free Association Books.

Smith, P. (1992). *The Emotional Labour of Nursing*. Basingstoke: Macmillan.

Speck, P. (1999). Working with dying people: On being good enough. In: A. Obholzer & V. Zagier Roberts (Eds.), *The Unconscious at Work: Individual and Organisational Stress in the Human Service*. London: Routledge.

Spence, D. P. (1983). *Narrative Truth and Historical Truth: Meaning and Interpretation in Psychoanalysis*. New York: W. W. Norton.

Spence, D. P. (1994). The special nature of clinical facts. *International Journal of Psychoanalysis, 75* (5/6): 915–927.

Steinbeck, J. E. (1937). *Of Mice and Men*. London: Penguin.

Steiner, J. (1982). Perverse relationships between parts of the self: A clinical illustration. *International Journal of Psychoanalysis, 63*: 241–251.

Stern, D. N. (1985a). *The Interpersonal World of the Infant*. New York: Basic Books.

Stern, D. N. (1985b). The sense of an emergent self. In: *The Interpersonal World of the Infant* (pp. 37–68). London : Karnac.

Stokes, J. (1994). The unconscious at work in groups and teams. In: A. Obholzer & V. Zagier Roberts (Eds.), *The Unconscious at Work: Individual and Organisational Stress in the Human Service*. London: Routledge.

Strathern, M. (Ed.) (2000). *Audit Cultures: Anthropological Studies in Accounting, Ethics and the Academy*. London: Routledge.

Summerfield, D. (2000). Childhood, war, refugeedom and "trauma": Three core questions for mental health professionals. *Transcultural Psychiatry, 37*: 3.

Symington, J. (1985). The survival function of primitive omnipotence. *International Journal of Psycho-Analysis, 66*: 481–486.

TES (2002). *Times Educational Supplement,* 1 March, pp. 12–14.

Toulmin, S. (1972). *Human Understanding, Vol. 1: General Introduction and Part 1*. Princeton, NJ: Princeton University Press.

Travers, M. (2007). *The New Bureaucracy: Quality Assurance and Its Critics*. Bristol: Policy Press.

Waddell, M. (1998a). *Inside Lives: Psychoanalysis and the Growth of the Personality*. Tavistock Clinic Series. London: Karnac.

Waddell, M. (1998b). The scapegoat. In: R. Anderson & A. Dartington (Eds.), *Facing It Out: Clinical Perspectives on Adolescent Disturbance*. London: Duckworth.

Waddell, M. (2002). *Inside Lives: Psychoanalysis and the Growth of the Personality*. London: Karnac.

Warman, A., & Jackson, E. (2007). Recruiting and retaining children and families' social workers: The potential of work discussion groups. *Journal of Social Work Practice, 21* (1): 35–48.

Wells, G. (2000). Dialogic inquiry in education: Building on Vygotsky's legacy. In: C. D. Lee & P. Smagorinsky (Eds.), *Vygotskian Perspectives on Literacy Research* (pp. 51–85). New York: Cambridge University Press.

Whittaker, S., Hardy, G., Lewis, K., & Buchan, L. (2005). An exploration of psychological well-being with young Somali refugee and asylum-seeker women. *Clinical Child Psychology and Psychiatry, 10*: 2.

Williams, G. (1981). Psychic pain and psychic damage. In: S. Box, B. Copley, J. Magagna, & E. Moustaki (Eds.), *Psychotherapy with Families: An Analytic Approach* (pp. 93–104). London: Routledge & Kegan Paul.

Williams, G. (1997). On gang dynamics. In: *Internal Landscapes and Foreign Bodies: Eating Disorders and Other Pathologies*. London: Duckworth.

Williams, G., Williams, P., Desmarais, J., & Ravenscroft, K. (Eds.) (2004). *The Generosity of Acceptance, Vols. 1 & 2*. London: Karnac.

Winnicott, D. W. (1965). *The Maturational Processes and the Facilitating Environment*. London: Hogarth Press.

Winnicott, D. W. (1971). *Playing and Reality*. London & New York: Routledge/Tavistock.

Winnicott, D. W. (1975). The antisocial tendency. In: *Through Paediatrics to Psychoanalysis*. London: Hogarth Press.

Winnicott, D. W. (1984). *Deprivation and Delinquency*. London, Tavistock.

Youell, B. (2006). *The Learning Relationship*. Tavistock Clinic Series. London: Karnac.

INDEX

For Product Safety Concerns and Information please contact our EU representative GPSR@taylorandfrancis.com
Taylor & Francis Verlag GmbH, Kaufingerstraße 24, 80331 München, Germany

www.ingramcontent.com/pod-product-compliance
Lightning Source LLC
Chambersburg PA
CBHW060741150926
51501CB00003B/65

* 9 7 8 0 3 6 7 3 2 9 8 5 3 *